The Comprehensive Guide to Plant-Based Lunch

Learn Everything You Need to Know About Plant-Based Lunch and Boost Your Diet

I0145981

Carl Brady

Table of contents

Lentil Tabouli Salad

Preparation time: 5 minutes Cooking time: 15 minutes Servings: 4

Ingredients:

For the Salad: 1 1/2 cups puy lentils, cooked 1/3 cup diced red onion 2 cups diced tomatoes 1/4 cup chopped mint 1 1/2 cups chopped parsley

For the Dressing: 1/3 teaspoon ground black pepper 1 teaspoon cinnamon 1 teaspoon salt 2 teaspoon allspice 3 tablespoons olive oil 1 lemon, juiced, zested

Directions: Prepare the dressing and for this, place all of its ingredients in a small bowl and whisk until smooth. Take a large bowl, place all the ingredients for the salad in it, top with prepared dressing and toss until well coated. Let the salad stand for 10 minutes and then serve

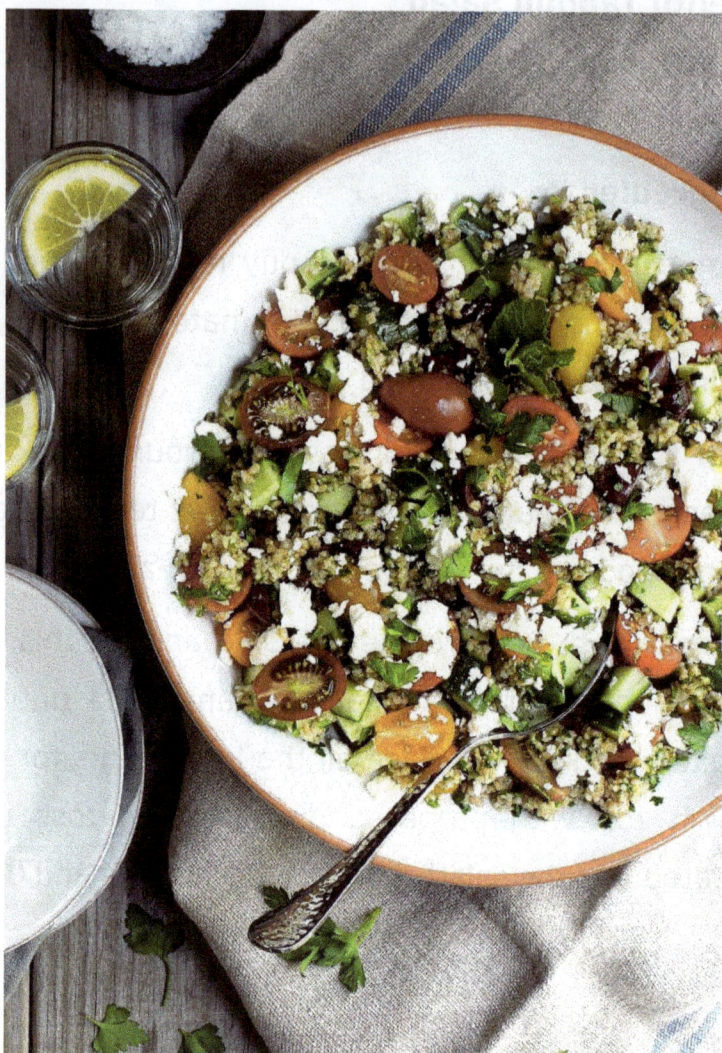

Moroccan Salad with Blood Oranges

Preparation time: 15 minutes Cooking time: 0 minute Servings: 4

Ingredients:

1 cup quinoa, cooked 3 blood oranges, divided 2 green onions, sliced ¼ cup sliced kalamata olives ¼ teaspoon salt ¼ teaspoon ground black pepper 1 tablespoon apple cider vinegar ¼ cup olive oil 1 teaspoon honey ¼ cup slivered almonds, toasted 12 mint leaves, torn

Directions:

Take a large bowl, place all the ingredients in it, except the last two ones, and toss until well coated. Top the salad with almonds and mint and then serve straight away.

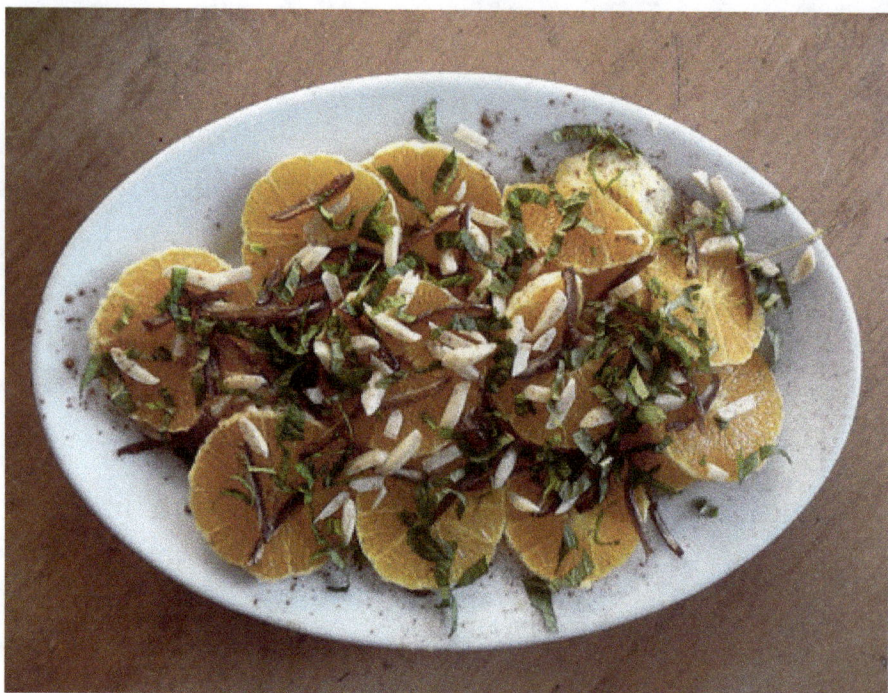

Cucumber Salad with Chili and Lime

Preparation time: 5 minutes Cooking time: 0 minute
Servings: 4

Ingredients:

1 jalapeno, deseeded, diced

2 large cucumbers, sliced

¼ of a medium red onion, sliced

½ bunch of cilantro

½ teaspoon red chili flakes

1/2 teaspoon salt

½ teaspoon coriander

3 tablespoons lime juice

2 tablespoons olive oil

Directions:

Take a large bowl, place all the ingredients in it, and toss until well coated. Serve straight away

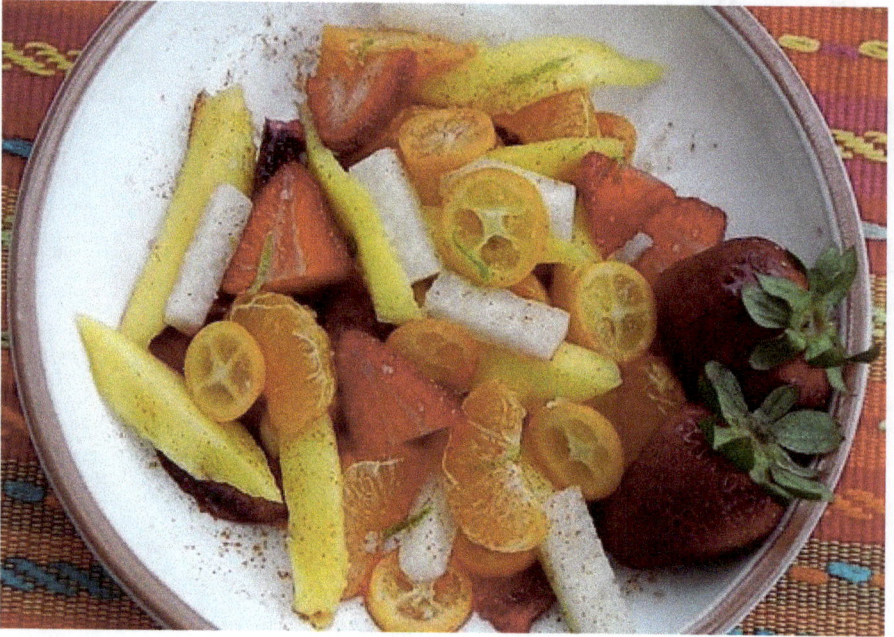

Lemon & Strawberry Soup

Preparation Time:4 hours and 10 minutes Cooking Time:0 minuteServings: 4

Ingredients:

1 cup buttermilk

3 cups strawberries, sliced

1 tsp. lemon thyme

2 tsp. lemon zest

2 tbsp. honey

Directions:

Blend the buttermilk and strawberries in your food processor. Transfer this mixture to a bowl. Add the thyme and lemon zest. Chill in the refrigerator for 4 hours. Strain the soup and stir in the honey. Serve in bowls.

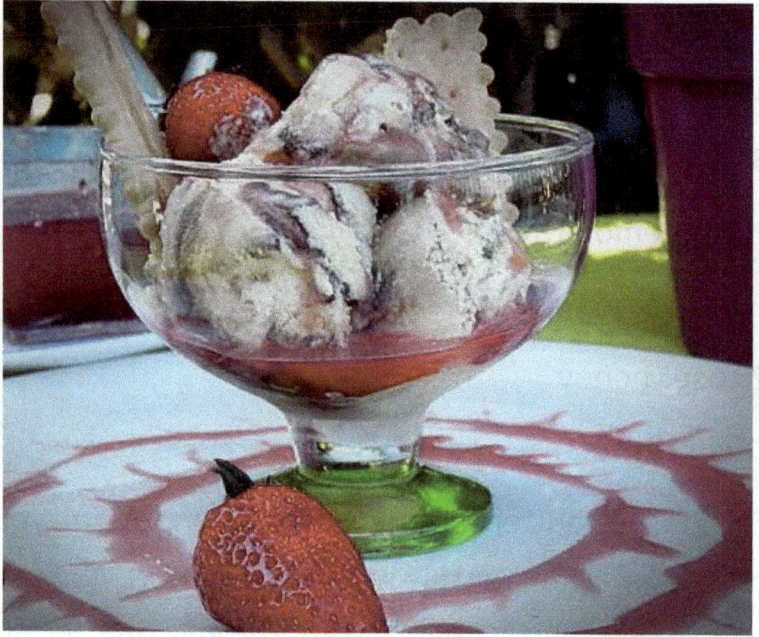

Bursting Black Bean Soup

Servings: 6 Preparation time: 8 hours and 10 minutes

Ingredients:

1 pound of black beans, uncooked 1/4 cup of lentils, uncooked 1 medium-sized carrot, peeled and chopped 2 medium-sized green bell peppers, cored and chopped 1 stalk of celery, chopped 28 ounce of diced tomatoes 2 jalapeno pepper, seeded and minced 1 large red onion, peeled and chopped 3 teaspoons of minced garlic 1 tablespoon of salt 1/2 teaspoon ground black pepper 2 tablespoons of red chili powder 2 teaspoons of ground cumin 1/2 teaspoon of dried oregano 3 tablespoons of apple cider vinegar 1/2 cup of brown rice, uncooked 3 quarts of water, divided

Directions:

Place a large pot over medium-high heat, add the beans, pour in 1 1/2 quarts of water and boil it. Let it boil for 10 minutes, then remove the pot from the heat, let it stand for 1 hour and then cover the pot. Drain the beans and add it to a 6-quarts slow cooker. Pour in the remaining 1 1/2 quarts of water and cover it with the lid. Plug in the slow cooker and let it cook for 3 hours at the high setting or until it gets soft. When the beans are done, add the remaining ingredients except for the rice and continue cooking for 3 hours on the low heat setting. When it is30 minutes left to finish, add the rice to the slow cooker and let it cook. When done, using an immersion blender process half of the soup and then serve.

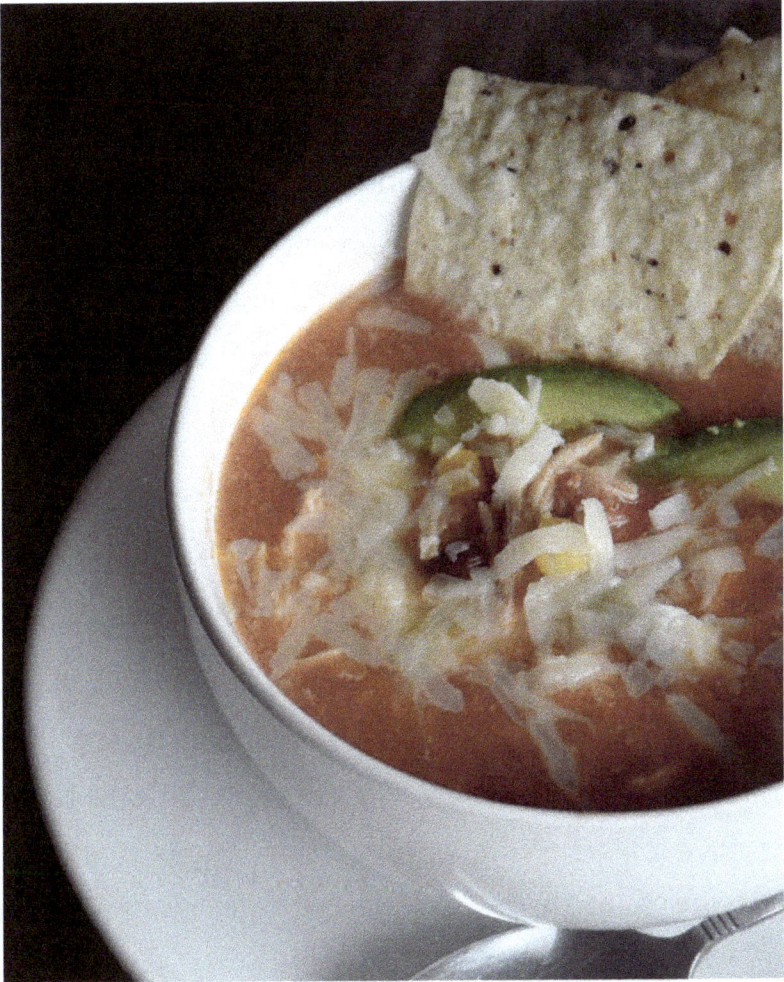

Portobello Onion Burgers

Preparation time: 10 minutes Cooking time: 30 minutes
Servings 2 burgers

Ingredients:

1 large green onion, cut into rings 2 tablespoons olive oil
2 Portobello mushrooms 1 teaspoon balsamic vinegar 1/8
teaspoon chili flakes 1 teaspoon agave syrup 1 teaspoon
soy sauce Salt, pepper (to taste)

Directions:

Add one tablespoon of olive oil to frying pan and heat
over low. Sauté onions for approximately 20 minutes,
until tender. After cooked, add chili flakes. In a large
mixing bowl, create a sauce by combining soy sauce,
balsamic vinegar, agave syrup, and salt/pepper. Coat the
mushrooms evenly with this sauce. Add one tablespoon
of olive oil to frying pan and heat over medium. Cook
burgers on each side 7 minutes, until golden brown.

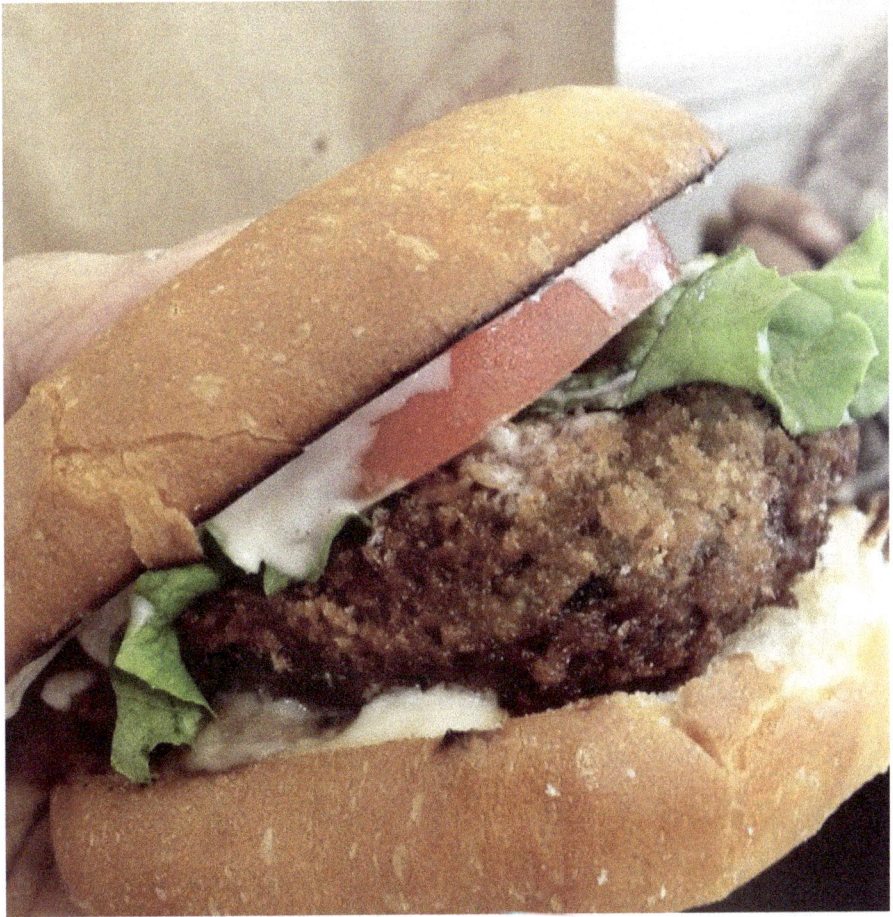

Tofu Almond Burgers

Preparation time: 10 minutes Cooking time: 30 minutes Servings 6–8 burgers

Ingredients:

2 tablespoons flax seeds, freshly ground 4 tablespoons water 1 package firm tofu, crumbled 1 carrot, peeled and grated 2 green onions, finely chopped 2 tablespoons sesame oil 1 teaspoon grated ginger 2 garlic cloves, minced 2/3 cup slivered almonds, toasted 2 teaspoons soy sauce 1 tablespoon sesame seeds

Directions:

In a small mixing bowl, combine flax seed and water. Pour sesame oil in a large skillet and warm on low heat. Sauté green onion, carrot, garlic and ginger for 4–5 minutes, until tender. In a large mixing bowl, add remaining ingredient list, flax seed mixture, sautéed items and combine. Using wet hands, form the mixture into a burger shape. Add one tablespoon of olive oil to frying pan and heat over medium. Cook burgers on each side 6 minutes, until golden brown.

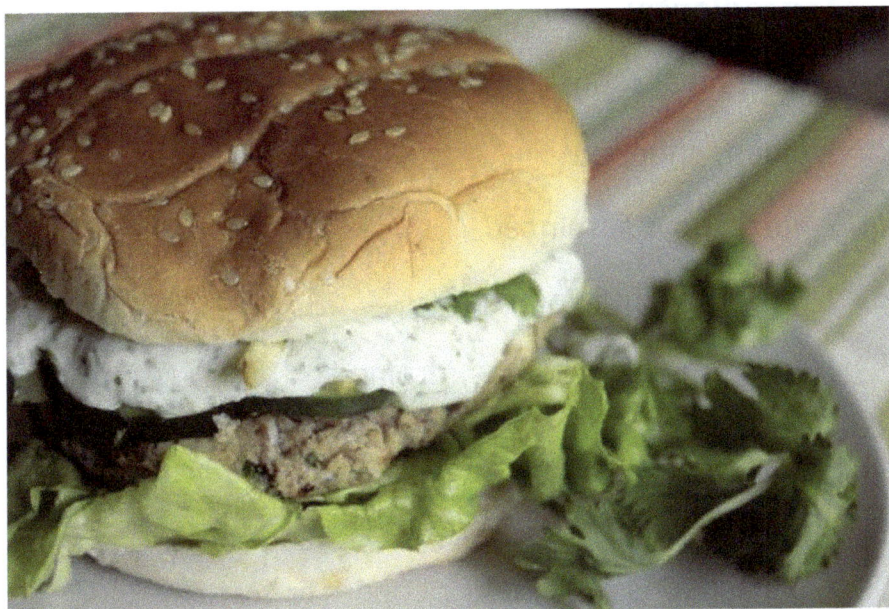

Mushroom Chickpea Burgers

Preparation time: 10 minutes Cooking time: 50 minutes
Servings 6–8 burgers

Ingredients:

2 cups mushrooms, finely chopped

1 onion, chopped

2 garlic cloves, minced

1 teaspoon curry powder

1 cup canned chickpeas, drained

2 carrots, peeled and grated

2 tablespoons chopped coriander

2 tablespoons flour Salt, pepper (to taste)

Directions:

In a medium size frying pan, heat one tablespoon of olive
oil and sauté onion and garlic for approximately 2
minutes. Add curry, carrots and mushrooms, turn heat

down to low and continue to cook for ten minutes. Set aside. In a food processor, pulse the chickpeas until a paste forms. In a large mixing bowl, combine the mushroom mixture an the paste. Stir in coriander, flour, and salt/pepper. Wet your hands and mold mixture into a burger shape. Add one tablespoon of olive oil to a frying pan on medium heat. Burger will be cooked thoroughly when both sides are a golden brown. Serve on your favorite bread, using toppings of your choice and tastiest condiments.

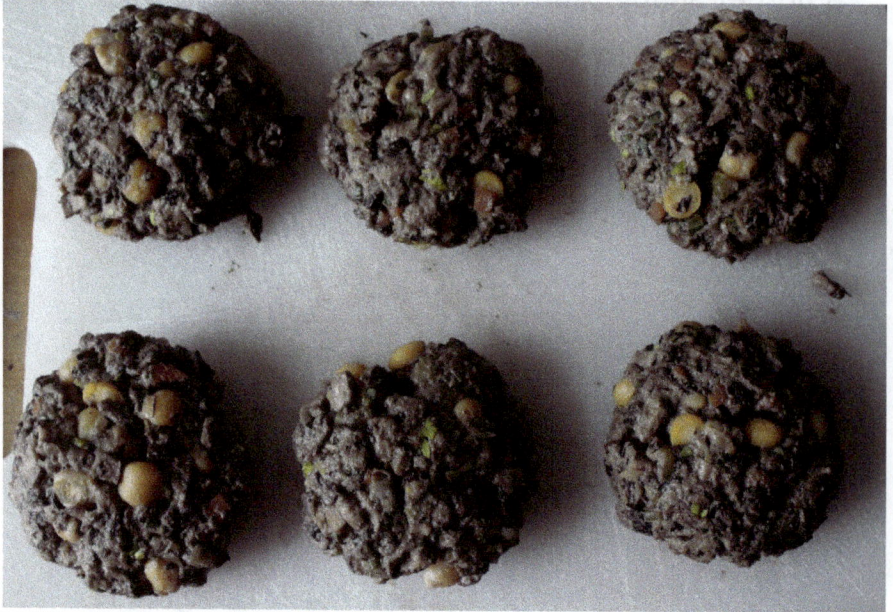

Summer Chickpea Salad

Serves: 4 Preparation Time: 15 Minutes

Ingredients:

1 ½ Cups Cherry Tomatoes, Halved

1 Cup English Cucumber, Slices

1 Cup Chickpeas, Canned, Unsalted, Drained & Rinsed

¼ Cup Red Onion, Slivered

2 Tablespoon Olive Oil

1 ½ Tablespoons Lemon Juice, Fresh

1 ½ Tablespoons Lemon Juice, Fresh Sea

Salt & Black Pepper to Taste

Directions: Mix everything together, and toss to combine before serving.

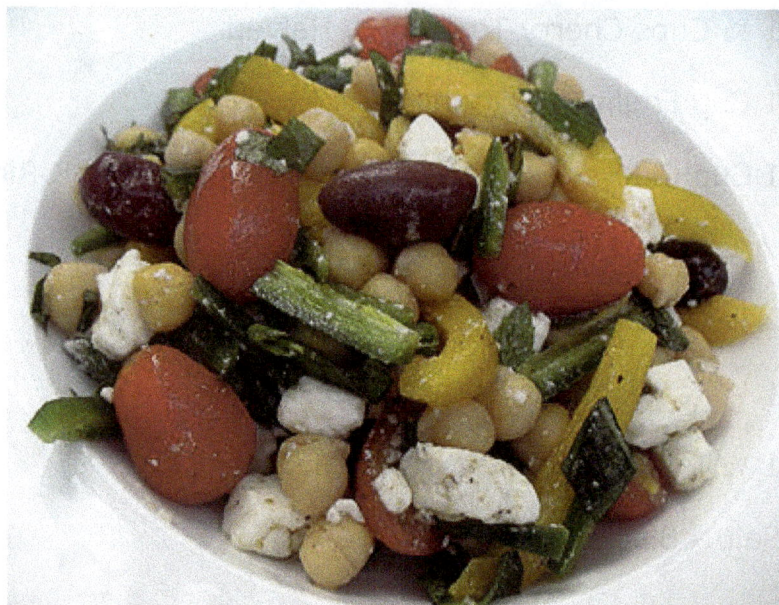

Fruity Kale Salad

Serves: 4 Preparation Time: 30 Minutes

Ingredients:

Salad: 10 Ounces Baby Kale ½ Cup Pomegranate Arils 1 Tablespoon Olive Oil 1 Apple, Sliced Dressing: 3 Tablespoons Apple Cider Vinegar 3 Tablespoons Olive Oil 1 Tablespoon Tahini Sauce (Optional) Sea Salt & Black Pepper to Taste

Directions:

Wash and dry the kale. If kale is too expensive, you can also use lettuce, arugula or spinach. Take the stems out, and chop it. Combine all of your salad ingredients together. Combine all of your dressing ingredients together before drizzling it over the salad to serve.

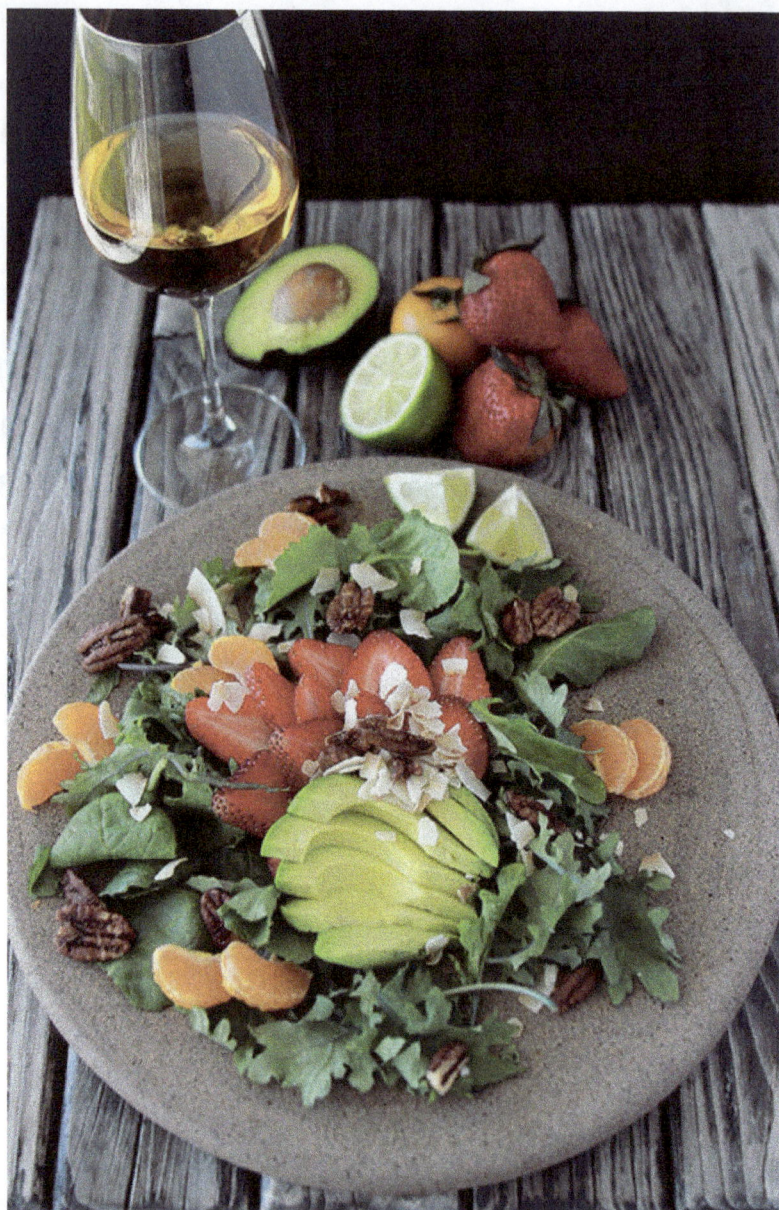

Avocado & Radish Salad

Serves: 2 Preparation Time: 10 Minutes

Ingredients:

1 Avocado, Sliced 6 Radishes, Sliced 2 Tomatoes, Sliced 1 Lettuce Head, Leaves Separated ½ Red Onion, Peeled & Sliced Dressing: ½ Cup Olive Oil ¼ Cup Lime Juice, Fresh ¼ Cup Apple Cider Vinegar 3 Cloves Garlic, Chopped Fine Sea Salt & Black Pepper to Taste

Directions:

Spread your lettuce leaves on a platter, and then layer with your onion, tomatoes, avocado and radishes. Whisk your dressing ingredients together before drizzling it over your salad. Interesting Facts: Avocados themselves are ranked within the top five of the healthiest foods on the planet, so you know that the oil that is produced from them is too. It is loaded with healthy fats and essential fatty acids. Like race bran oil it is perfect to cook with as well! Bonus: Helps in the prevention of diabetes and lowers cholesterol levels.

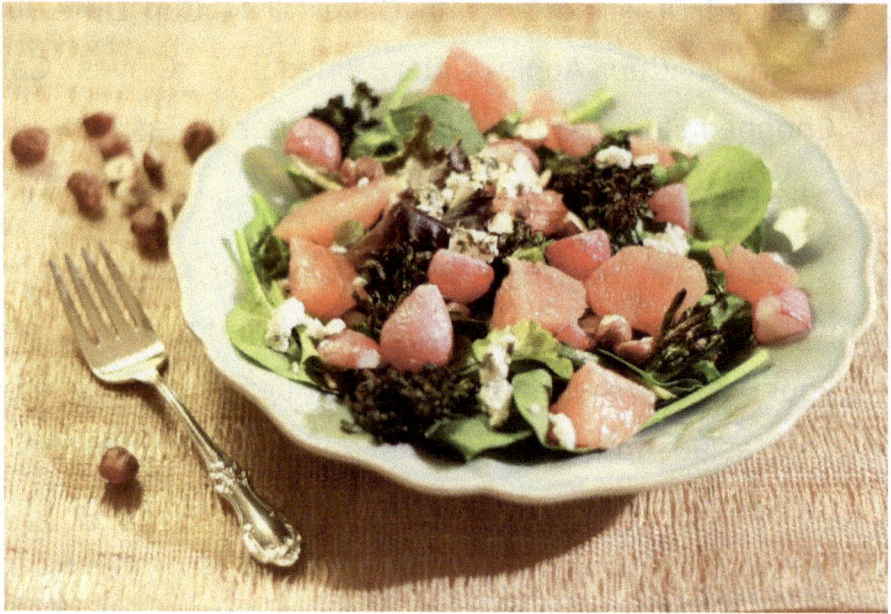

Watercress & Blood Orange

Salad Serves: 4 Preparation Time: 10 Minutes

Ingredients:

1 Tablespoon Hazelnuts, Toasted & Chopped 2 Blood Oranges (or Navel Oranges) 3 Cups watercress, Stems Removed 1/8 Teaspoon Sea Salt, Fine 1 Tablespoon Lemon Juice, Fresh 1 Tablespoon Honey, Raw 1 Tablespoon Water 2 Tablespoons Chives, Fresh

Directions:

Whisk your oil, honey, lemon juice, chives, salt and water together. Add in your watercress, tossing until it's coated. Arrange the mixture onto salad plates, and top with orange slices. Drizzle with remaining liquid, and sprinkle with hazelnuts. Interesting Facts: Lemons are popularly known as harboring loads of Vitamin C, but are also excellent sources of folate, fiber, and antioxidants. Bonus: Helps lower cholesterol. Double Bonus: Reduces risk of cancer and high blood pressure.

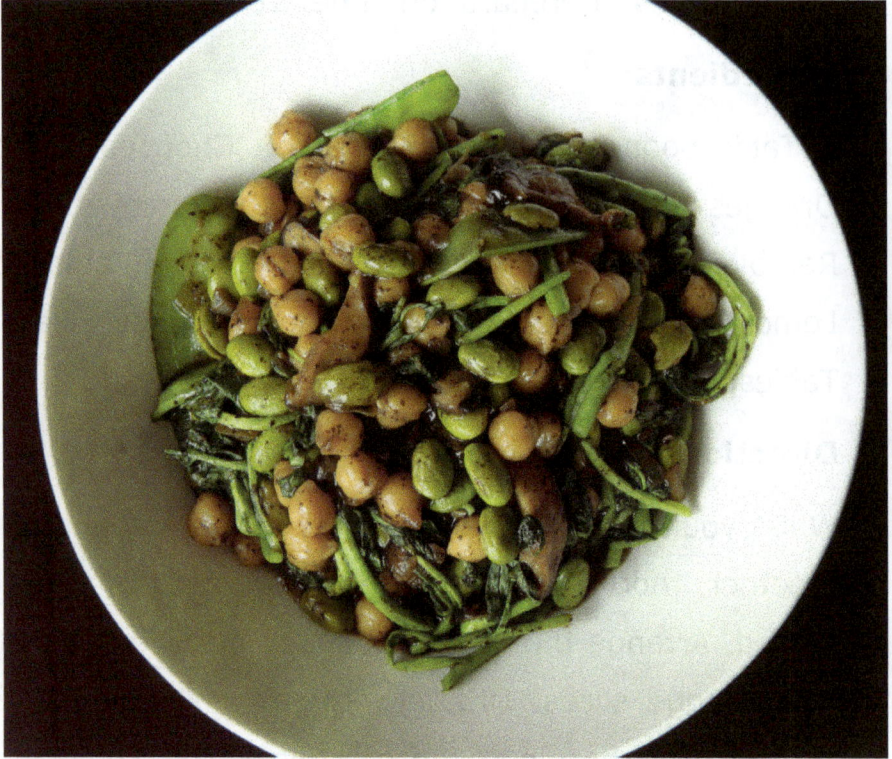

Tzatziki

Preparation Time: 20minutes

Ingredients:

1 cup of natural vegan yogurt 1/4 cucumber (grated) 1 tablespoon of fresh dill 1 teaspoon of lemon peel 1 tablespoon of Nutritional yeast 1 tsp black pepper 1 teaspoon of salt 1 chopped clove of garlic 1 tablespoon of olive oil 1 tablespoon of lemon juice

Directions: Preparation Mix all INGREDIENTS in a medium bowl. Stir together. Place on a serving plate, cover well and refrigerate up to 1 hour before serving.

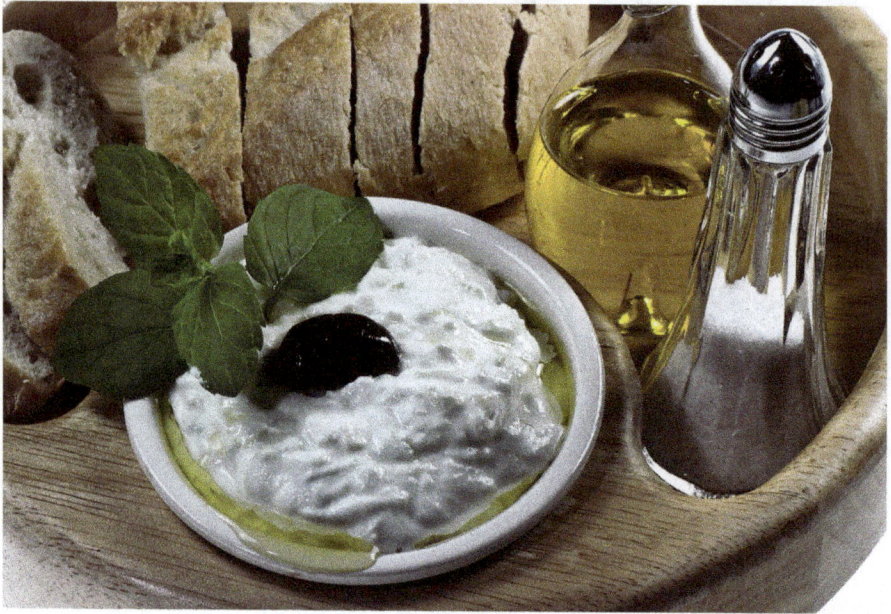

Fish sauce

Preparation Time: 30minutes

Ingredients:

1/2 cup grated wakame (see notes) 2 cups of filtered water 2 large cloves of garlic, crushed 1 teaspoon of whole peppercorns 1/3 cup of dark soy sauce with mushroom flavor, normal soy sauce or gluten-free tamari 1 teaspoon of Genmai Miso (it's quite salty, so optional)

Directions:

Combine the wakame, garlic, peppercorns and water in a large pan and cook. Lower the heat and simmer for about twenty minutes. Strain and return the liquid to the pot. Add the soy sauce, cook again and cook until the mixture is almost salty and unbearable. Remove from the heat and add miso. Transfer to a bottle and keep in the fridge. Use one by one to replace fish sauce in vegan recipes.

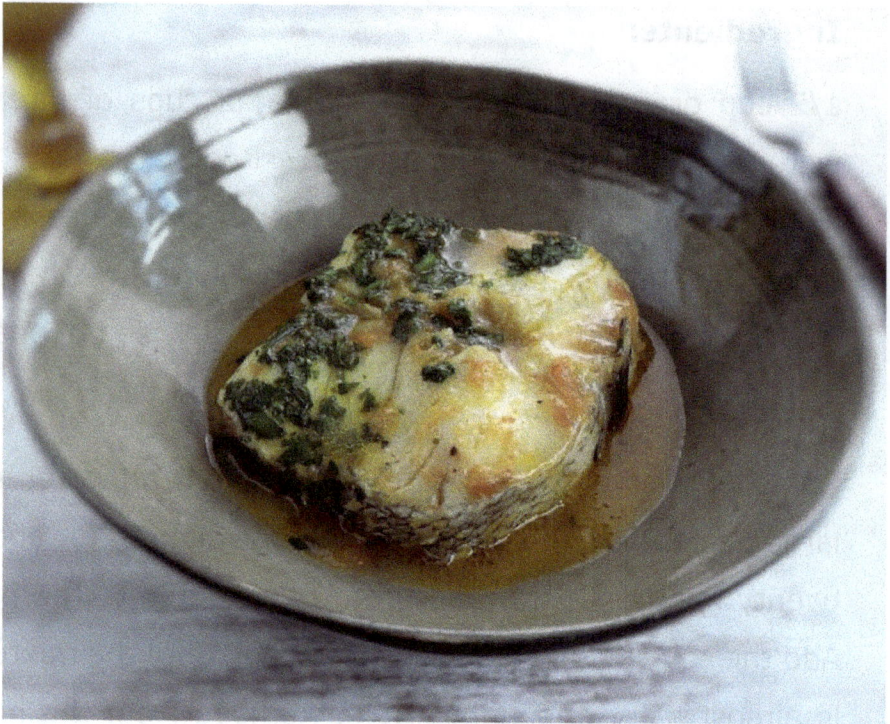

Creamy cucumber herb

Preparation Time: 10minutes

Ingredients:

3 ounces of cashew nuts, soaked in water for 2 hours 2 1/2 ounces of cucumber, peeled and chopped 1/4 cup of unsweetened milk 1/2 ounce chopped shallot 1/2 lemon juice 1 small clove of garlic, peeled 1 teaspoon of apple cider vinegar 1/2 teaspoon of salt 1/4 tsp garlic powder A pinch of ground black pepper 1 tablespoon of finely chopped fresh dill 1 tablespoon of finely chopped fresh parsley 1 tablespoon of finely chopped fresh chives

Directions:

Add all the INGREDIENTS except herbs in a small blender and mix to a creamy and smooth consistency. Add the herbs and mix well.

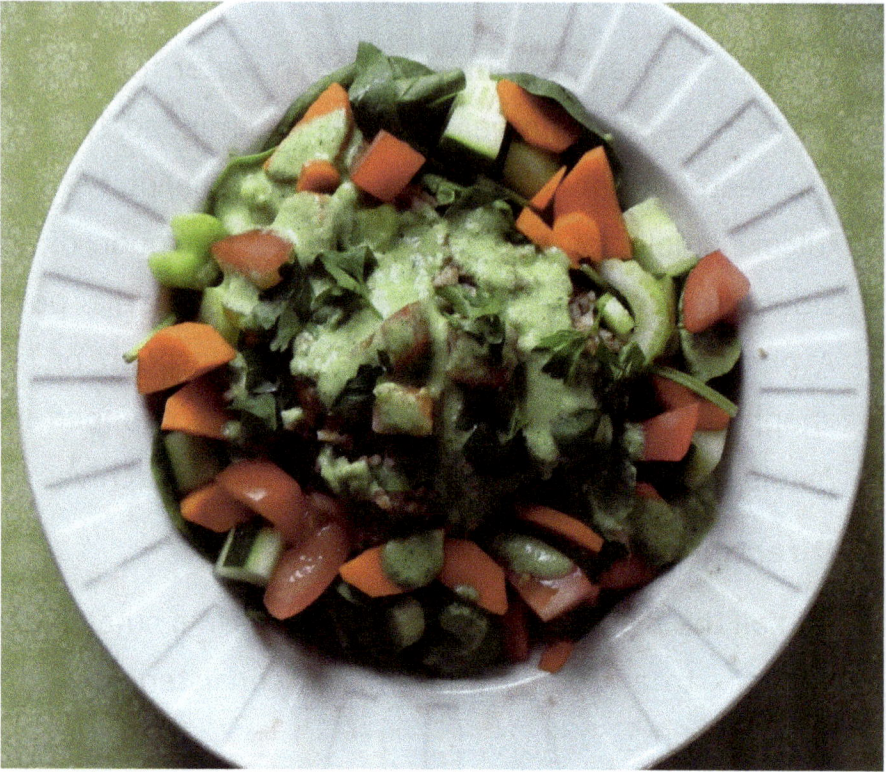

Roasted Vegetables in Balsamic Sauce

Preparation Time: 10 minutes Cooking Time: 23 minutes

Servings: 12

Ingredients:

1 onion, sliced into wedges 2 cloves garlic, minced 1 lb. green beans, trimmed 2 tablespoons olive oil Salt and pepper to taste 4 yellow summer squash, sliced ⅔ cup balsamic vinegar

Directions:

Preheat your oven to 450 degrees F. Toss onion, garlic and beans in olive oil. Transfer to a baking pan. Season with salt and pepper. Roast in the oven for 8 minutes. Add the squash. Roast for another 5 minutes. Transfer roasted vegetables in a food container. Reheat the veggies and toss in balsamic vinegar sauce when ready to serve.

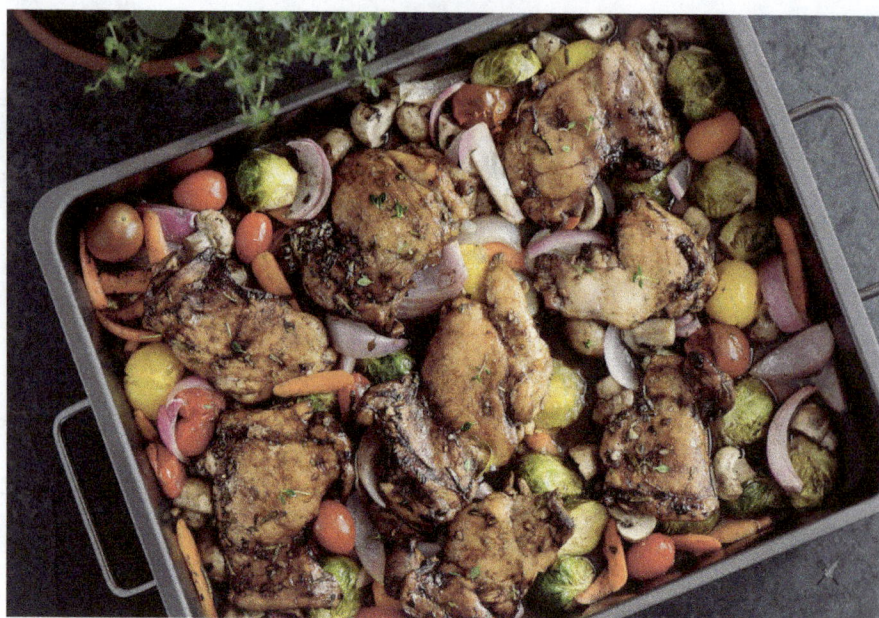

Vegetable Salad in Mason Jar

Preparation Time: 5 minutes Cooking Time: 0 minute Servings: 1

Ingredients:

2 tablespoons cashew sauce (recipe in the sauce section) 1 cup tofu cubes, roasted 1 tablespoon pumpkin seeds 1 cup carrots, roasted 2 cups mixed greens

Directions:

In a glass jar, layer the cashew sauce, tofu, seeds, carrots and mixed greens. Seal the jar. Refrigerate up to 5 days. Serve whenever ready to eat.

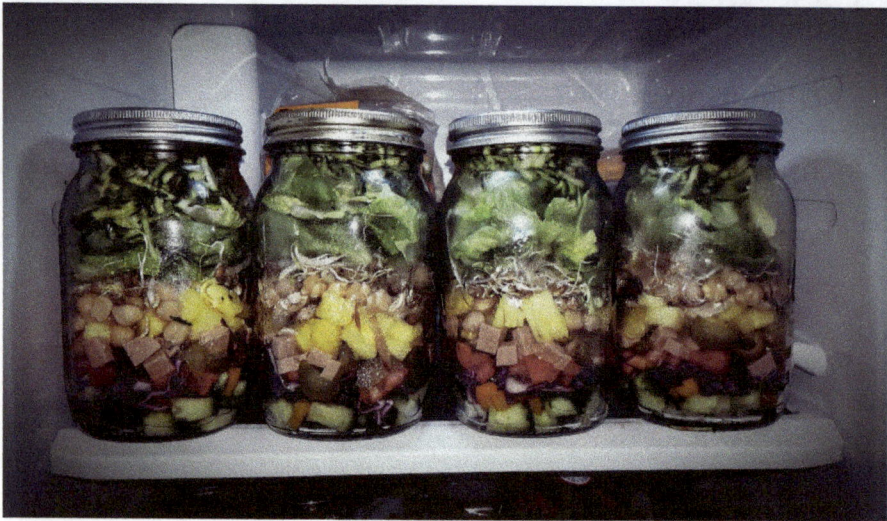

Mixed herbs with almonds and pepita pesto

Preparation Time: 30minutes

Ingredients:

1 cup wrapped fresh basil leaves 1 cup wrapped arugula 2 cloves garlic (grated) 1/2 cup raw pepita 1/4 cup raw almonds 1/4 cup fresh lemon juice 2 tbsp virgin olive oil 1/2 tsp salt (or to taste) 1/8 teaspoon pepper (or to taste) 2-3 tbsp of thin water

Directions:

Place all INGREDIENTS except olive oil and water in a food processor. Processing Before combining, split sides as needed. Sprinkle olive oil on top while the machine is still running. This should work smoothly. Add Water 1 Ch. Simultaneously process after each addition and scroll through the pages as needed until you reach the desired consistency.

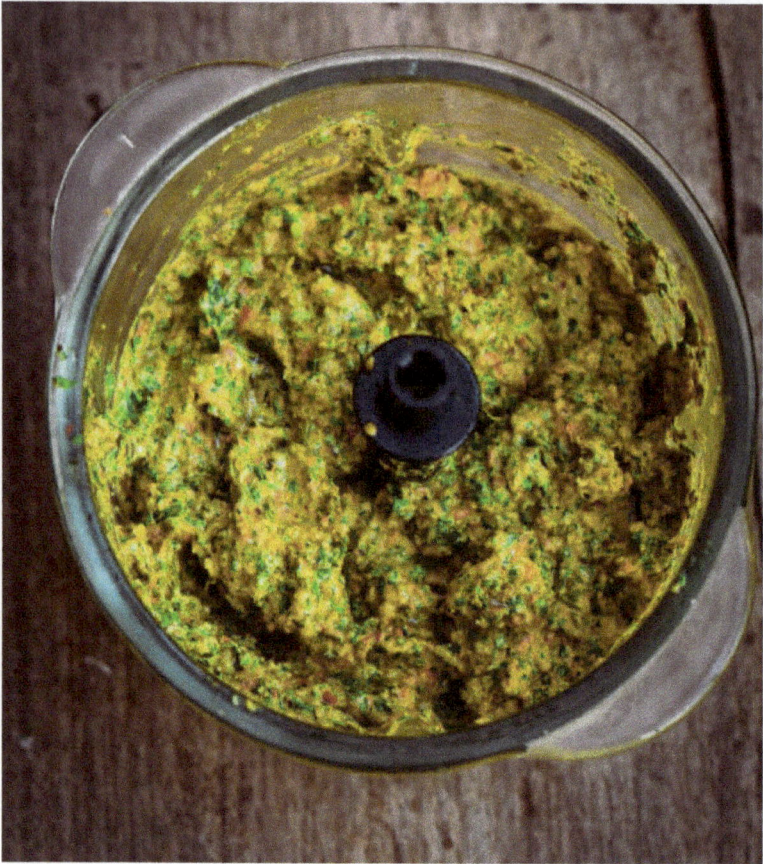

Diluited banana caramel sauce

Preparation Time: 30minutes

Ingredients:

2 large very ripe bananas 1/4 cup coconut sugar (use 1/2 cup if your banana is not too ripe or you like sweet sides) 2 tbsp brown rice syrup 1/2 cup milk milk 1 teaspoon pure vanilla extract 1/4 tsp salt

Directions:

Put all INGREDIENTS in a blender or food processor and puree for a few seconds until smooth. Pour the mixture into the baking sheet and bring to a boil. You may need to adjust the heat as it burns. You don't want to burn sugar, but you want a good bladder to reduce it. The mixture will be ready when it is reduced by about half.

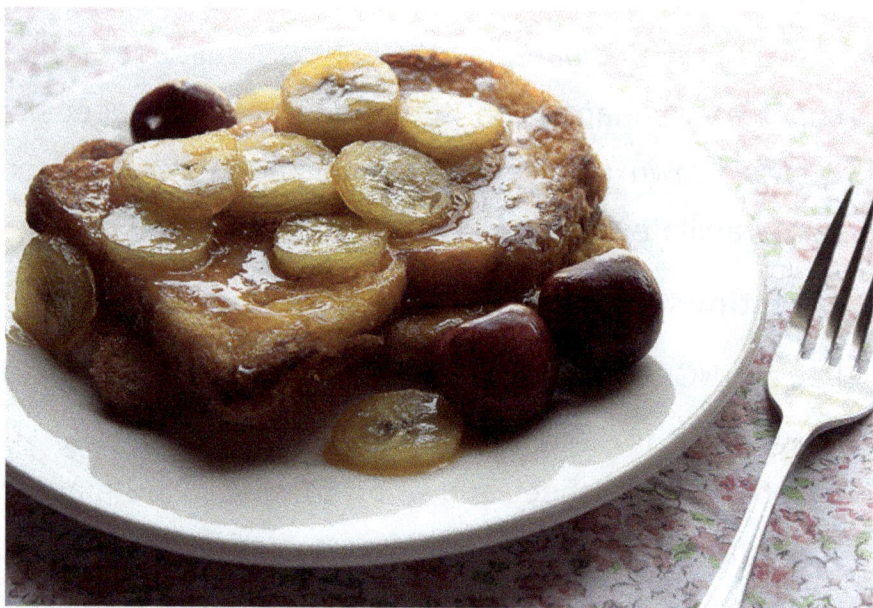

Zucchini Soup

Preparation Time: 5 minutes Cooking Time: 15 minutes

Servings: 4

Ingredients:

3 cups chicken broth 1 tbsp. tarragon, chopped 3 zucchinis, sliced 3 oz. cheddar cheese Salt and pepper to taste

Directions:

Pour the broth into a pot. Stir in the tarragon and zucchini. Bring to a boil and then simmer for 10 minutes. Transfer to a blender and blend until smooth. Put it back to the stove and stir in cheese. Season with salt and pepper.

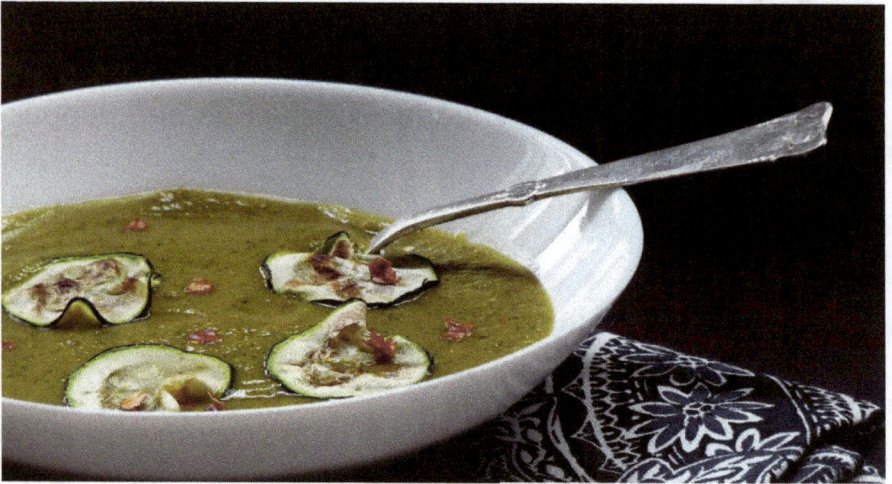

Corn & Black Bean Salad Salad: 6 Time: 10 Minutes

Ingredients:

¼ Cup Cilantro, Fresh & Chopped 1 Can Corn, Drained (10 Ounces) 1/8 Cup Red Onion, Chopped 1 Can Black Beans, Drained (15 Ounces) 1 Tomato, Chopped 3 Tablespoons Lemon Juice, Fresh 2 Tablespoons Olive Oil Sea Salt & Black Pepper to Taste

Directions:

Mix everything together, and then refrigerate until cool. Serve cold. Interesting Facts: Whole corn is a fantastic source of phosphorus, magnesium, and B vitamins. It also promotes healthy digestion and contains heart-healthy antioxidants. It is important to seek out organic corn in order to bypass all of the genetically modified product that is out on the market.

Red Pepper & Broccoli Salad

Serves: 2 Time: 15 Minutes Calories: 185 Protein: 4 Grams Fat: 14 Grams Carbs: 8 Grams

Ingredients:

Ounces Lettuce Salad Mix 1 Head Broccoli, Chopped into Florets 1 Red Pepper, Seeded & Chopped Dressing: 3 Tablespoons White Wine Vinegar 1 Teaspoon Dijon Mustard 1 Clove Garlic, Peeled & Chopped Fine ½ Teaspoon Black Pepper ½ Teaspoon Sea Salt, Fine 2 Tablespoons Olive Oil 1 Tablespoon Parsley, Chopped

Directions:

In boiling water, drain the broccoli it on a paper towel. Whisk together all dressing ingredients. Toss ingredients together before serving. Interesting Facts: This oil is the main source of dietary fat in a variety of diets. It contains many vitamins and minerals that play a part in reducing the risk of stroke and lowers cholesterol and high blood pressure and can also aid in weight loss. It is best consumed cold, as when it is heated it can lose some of its nutritive properties (although it is still great to cook with – extra virgin is best), many recommend taking a shot of cold oil olive daily! Bonus: if you don't like the taste or texture add a shot to your smoothie.

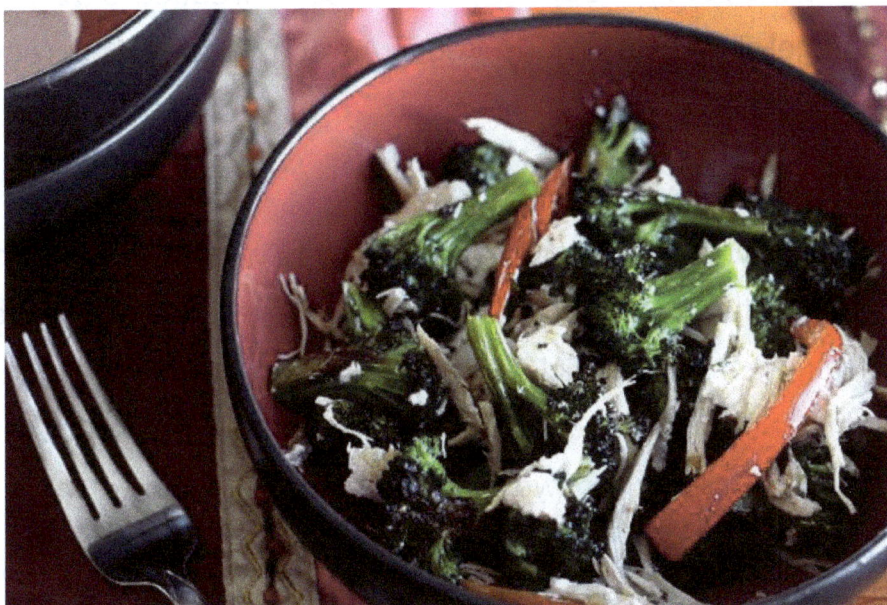

Cheesy Asparagus Pasta

Preparation time: 10 minutes Cooking time: 50 minutes Servings: 4

Ingredients:

2 Cups Pasta 1 Cup Vegan Cheese, Shredded 3 ½ Cups Vegetable Broth ½ Cup Vegan Alfredo Sauce 6 Asparagus Spears, Chopped

Directions:

Mix your pasta, broth and asparagus in your instant pot. Seal the lid, and cook on high pressure for seven minutes. Use a quick release, and rain your pasta. Add it all back into the cooker, and then stir in the sauce and cheese. Sauté for two minutes before serving warm.

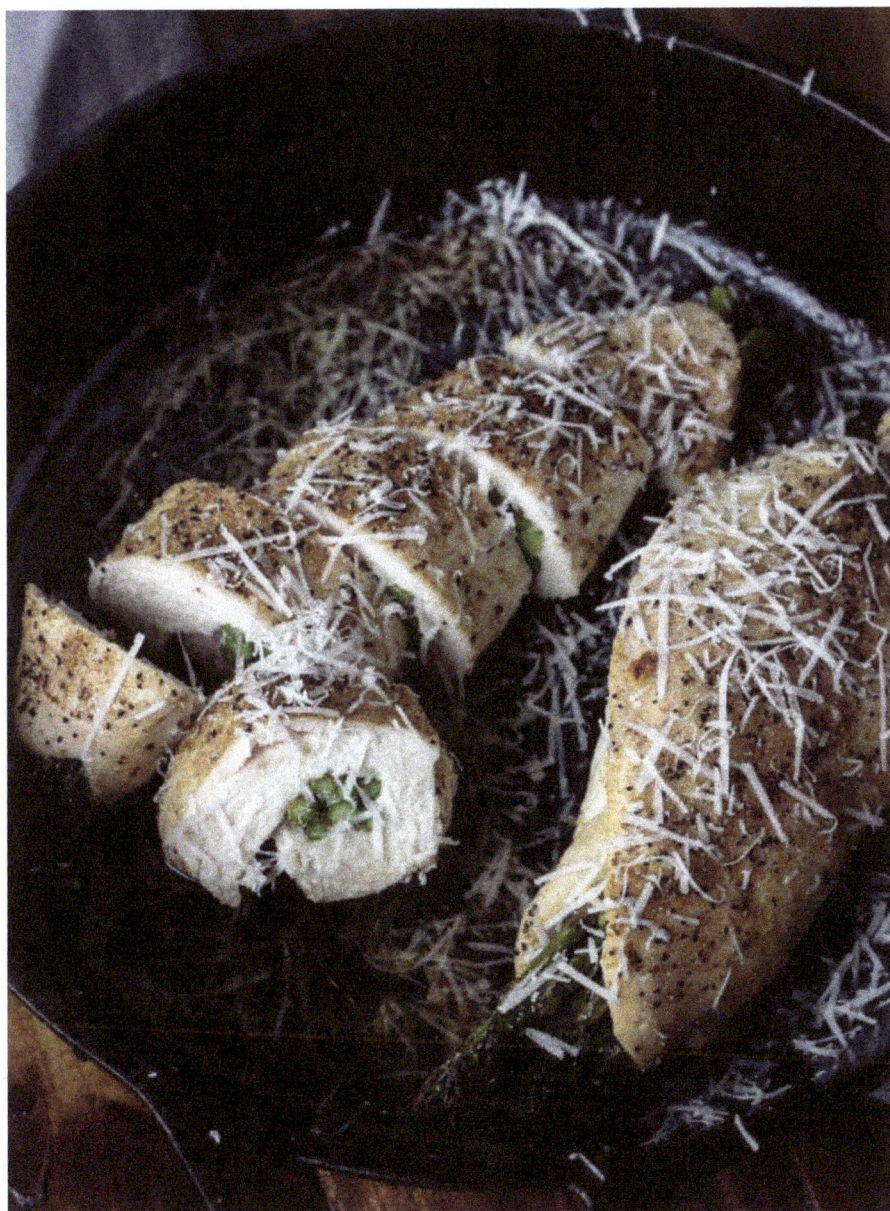

Kale & Mushroom Stroganoff

Preparation time: 10 minutes Cooking time: 40 minutes
Servings: 4

Ingredients:

1 Tablespoon Olive Oil 1 Sweet Onion, Diced 2 Cloves
Garlic, Minced 1 lb. Baby Bella Mushrooms, Sliced 1
Tomato, Diced 1 Teaspoon Smoked Paprika Sea Salt &
Black Pepper to Taste 1 Bay Leaf 3 Cups Campanella
Pasta 3 ¼ Cups Vegetable Stock 1 Cup Cashew Sour
Cream 3 Cups Kale, Rinsed & Torn

Directions: Press sauté and then add the oil. Once it's
hot cook the onion for two minutes, while stirring
frequently. Add the garlic, cooking for another minute
and stir well. Add the tomato, paprika, bay leaf,
mushrooms and salt. Allow it to sit for three minutes. Stir
in the pasta and stock, and then lock your lid. Cook on
high pressure for three minutes. Allow for a natural
pressure release for five minutes and then finish with a
quick release. Discard the bay leaf, and sauté for two
more minutes if there is excess liquid. Stir in the kale and
sour cream, allowing your kale to wilt for two minutes.
Season with salt before serving.

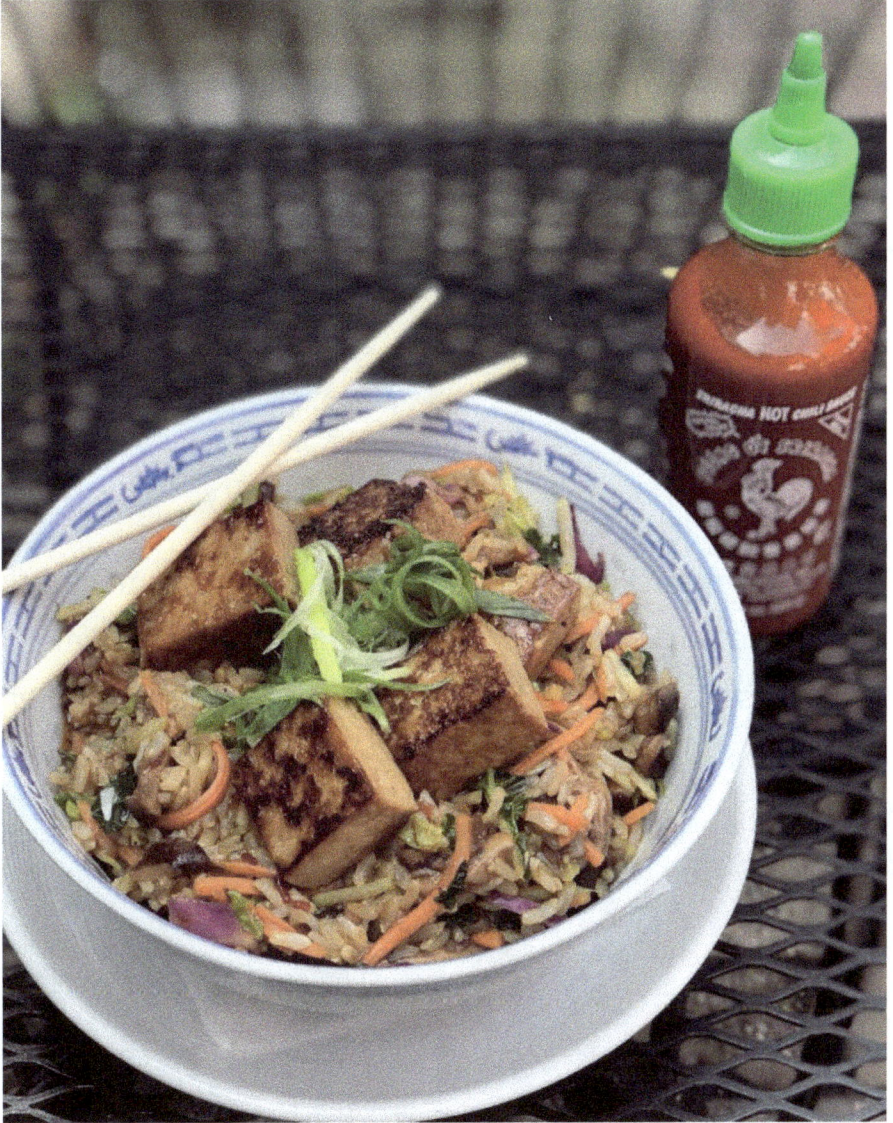

Edamame & Aleppo Pepper

Preparation Time: 5 minutes Cooking Time: 5 minutes

Serving: 1

Ingredients:

½ cup edamame pods Water

⅛ teaspoon Aleppo pepper

Directions: Place edamame pods in a steamer basket. Put the basket on top of a pot with water. Steam. Store in glass jar with lid. Season with Aleppo pepper before serving.

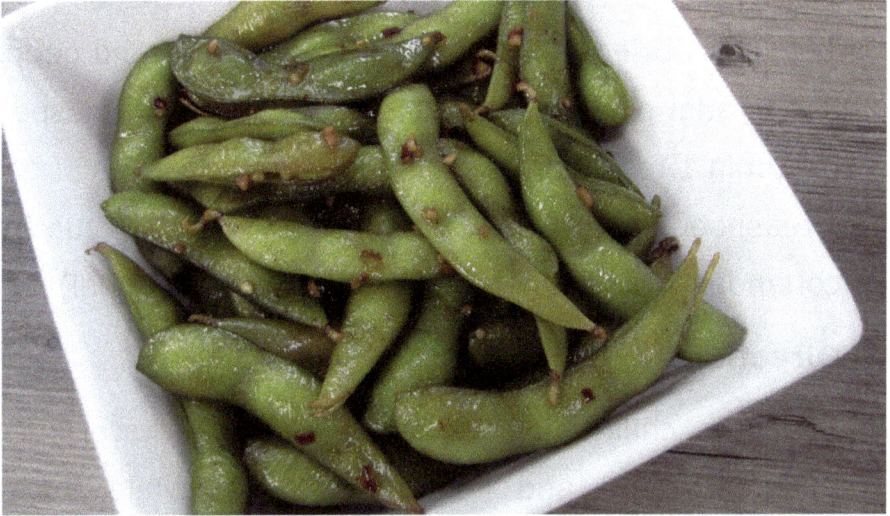

Harissa

Preparation Time: 30minutes

Ingredients:

1/4 cup of dried red cayenne pepper 20 soft red peppers like Byadgi or Wide Chili (also dried) 1 1/2 tablespoons of cumin 1 teaspoon of coriander seeds 4 cloves of garlic 1 teaspoon of salt 3 tablespoons of olive oil 1/4 cup fresh coriander 1 tablespoon of chopped mint (optional)

Directions:

Soak the chillies with 1/2 cup of warm water for 15 minutes. Drain and keep water. Meanwhile, roasted cumin and coriander. Grind the powder in a coffee grinder. Put the paprika, ground spices, garlic, salt and olive oil in a blender with a little water and cut into a paste. Add the chopped coriander and mint and press several times. Use a little more water if necessary. Store the mixture in the refrigerator then use as needed.

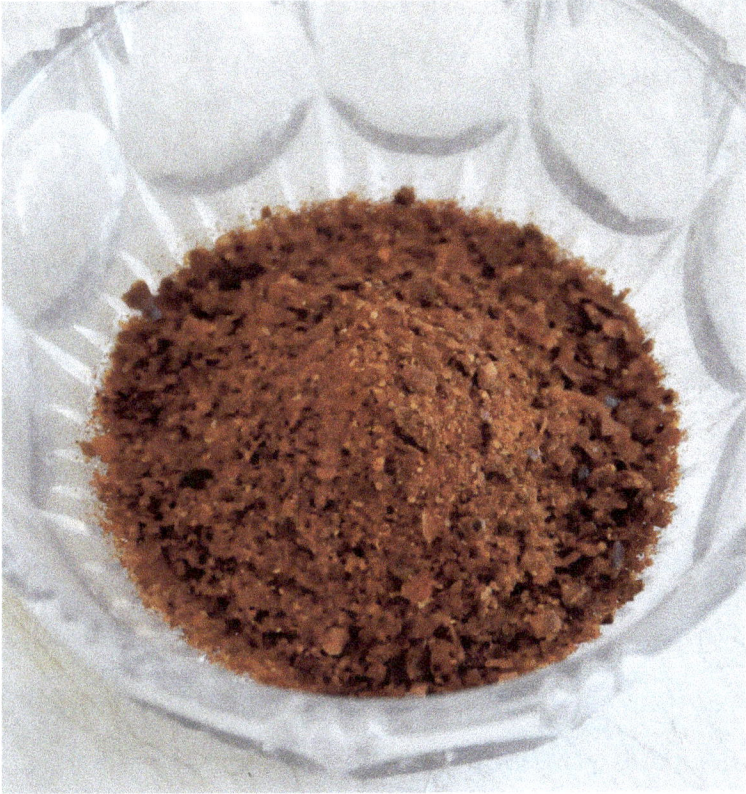

Toasted Banana Caramel Sauce

Preparation Time: 30minutes

Ingredients:

2 large ripe bananas 1/4 cup coconut sugar (use 1/2 cup if your bananas are not overripe or if you like sweeter things) 2 tbsp brown rice syrup 1/2 cup milk without milk 1 tsp pure vanilla extract 1/4 teaspoon salt

Directions:

Put all INGREDIENTS in a blender or food processor and beat for a few seconds until smooth. Pour the mixture into a pan and bring to a boil. Reduce heat and simmer for 20 minutes, stirring constantly. It may be necessary to adjust the heat as it boils. You don't want sugars to burn, but you want a good bubble to occur so that it shrinks. The mixture is ready when it is halved.

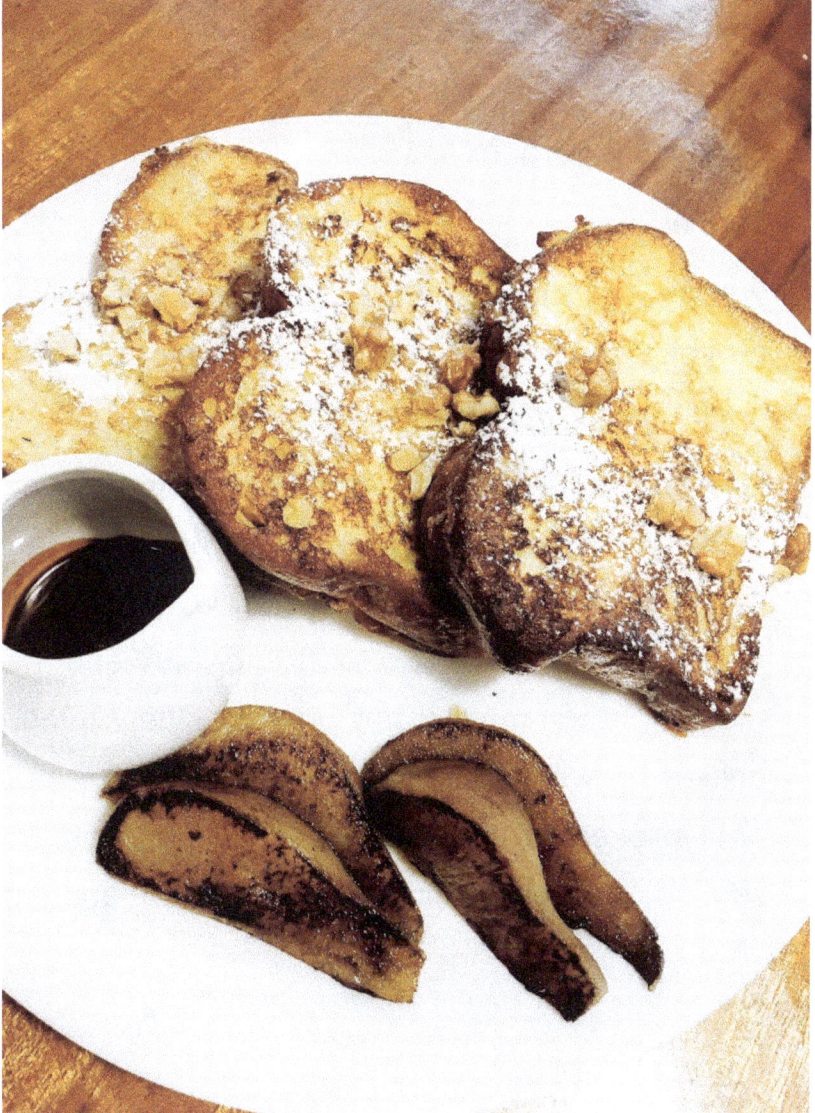

Mushroom Pineapple Burgers

Preparation time: 10 minutes Cooking time: 40 minutes Servings 2 burgers

Ingredients:

2 Portobello mushrooms 2 slices fresh pineapple 1/4 cup teriyaki sauce 1 teaspoon agave syrup Salt, pepper Vegan burger buns

Directions: Create a sauce by combining teriyaki sauce, agave syrup, and salt/pepper. Brush the sauce over mushrooms and pineapple, coating evenly. Add one tablespoon of olive oil to frying pan and heat over medium. Cook mushrooms on each side 7 minutes, until golden brown. Heat pineapple in pan with mushrooms until cooked through. Using the vegan burger bun for serving, layer mushrooms and pineapple and enjoy!

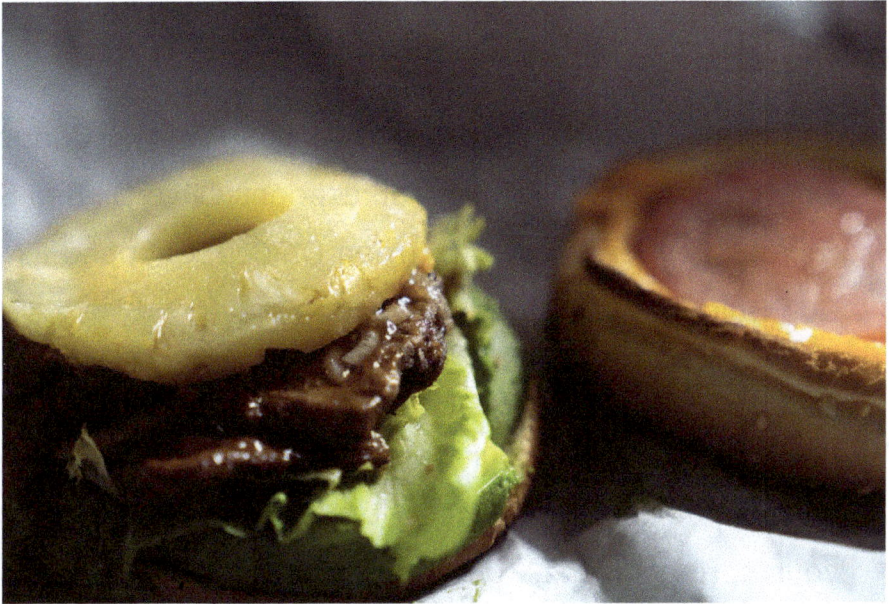

Parsley Salad

Serves: 8 Preparation Time: 30 Minutes

Ingredients:

3 Lemons, Juiced 150 Grams Flat Lea Parsley, Chopped Fine 1 Cup Boiled Water 5 Tablespoons Olive Oil Sea Salt & Black Pepper to Taste 6 Green Onions, Chopped Fine 1 Cup Bulgur 4 Tomatoes, Chopped Fine

Directions:

Add your Bulgur to your water, and mix well. Put a towel on top of it to steam it. Keep it to the side, and then chop your spring onions, tomatoes and parsley. Put them in your salad bowl. Pour your juice into the mixture, and then add in your olive oil, salt and pepper. Put this mixture over your bulgur to serve.

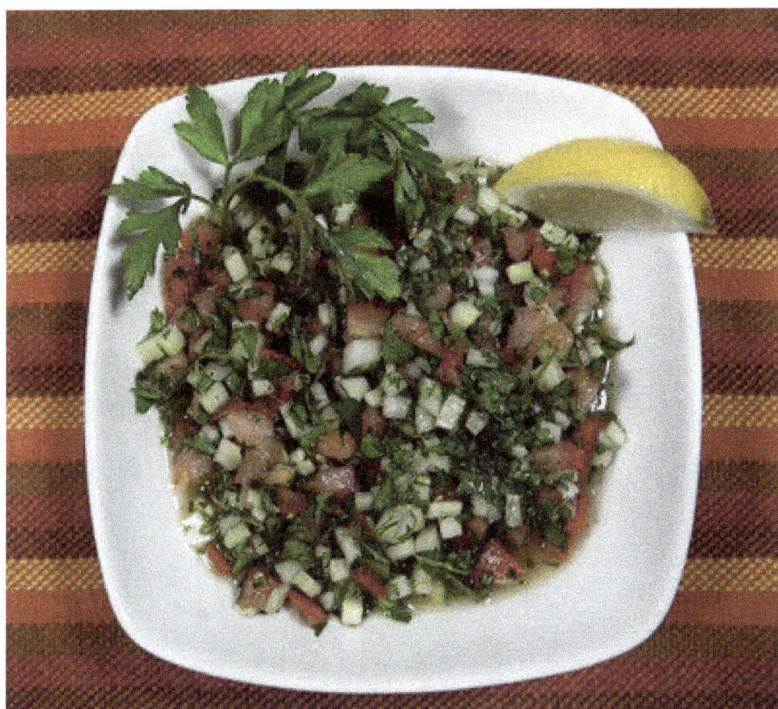

Cranberry and Quinoa Salad

Preparation time: 15 minutes Cooking time: 0 minute

Servings: 6

Ingredients:

2 cups cooked quinoa 1/4 cup chopped red onion 1/2 cup shredded carrots 1/2 cup dried cranberries 1/2 cup diced green bell pepper 4 tablespoons chopped cilantro 1 ½ teaspoon curry powder 2/3 teaspoon salt 1/3 teaspoon ground black pepper 1/8 teaspoon cumin 1/3 cup toasted sliced almonds 4 tablespoons pepitas Olive oil as needed for drizzling 1 lime, juiced Lime, sliced into wedges

Directions:

Place all the ingredients in a large bowl, toss until well combined and let the salad refrigerate for 15 minutes. Serve straight away.

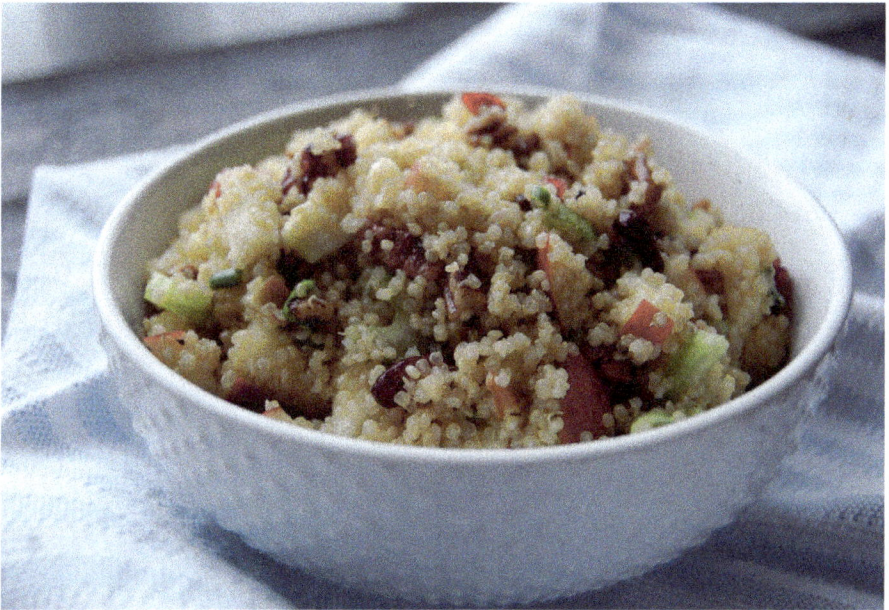

Cucumber Salad with Tofu

Preparation time: 10 minutes Cooking time: 10 minutes

Servings: 4

Ingredients:

2 large cucumbers, sliced ½ of medium green bell pepper, sliced into strips 14 ounces tofu, extra-firm, drained, cubed 3 green onions, chopped ½ of green chili pepper, deseeded, sliced into thin strips 3 large carrots, shaved into ribbons ¼ teaspoon salt 1/3 cup roasted almond slices 1/2 cup cilantro leaves and stem 1 tablespoon sesame oil

For the Dressing: 2 cloves of garlic, peeled 1-inch piece of ginger, grated ¼ teaspoon red pepper flakes 1 tablespoon soy sauce 2 tablespoons rice vinegar 1 teaspoon maple syrup 6 tablespoons sesame oil

Directions:

Fry tofu cubes in hot sesame oil over medium heat for 10 minutes until browned and then set aside. Meanwhile, sprinkle salt over cucumber slices, set aside for 10 minutes, then drain them, rinse them and pat dry with paper towels. Prepare the dressing, and for this, place all its ingredients in a food processor and process for 2 minutes until smooth. Place everything in a large bowl, toss until well coated, then top the salad with extra nuts and green onions and serve.

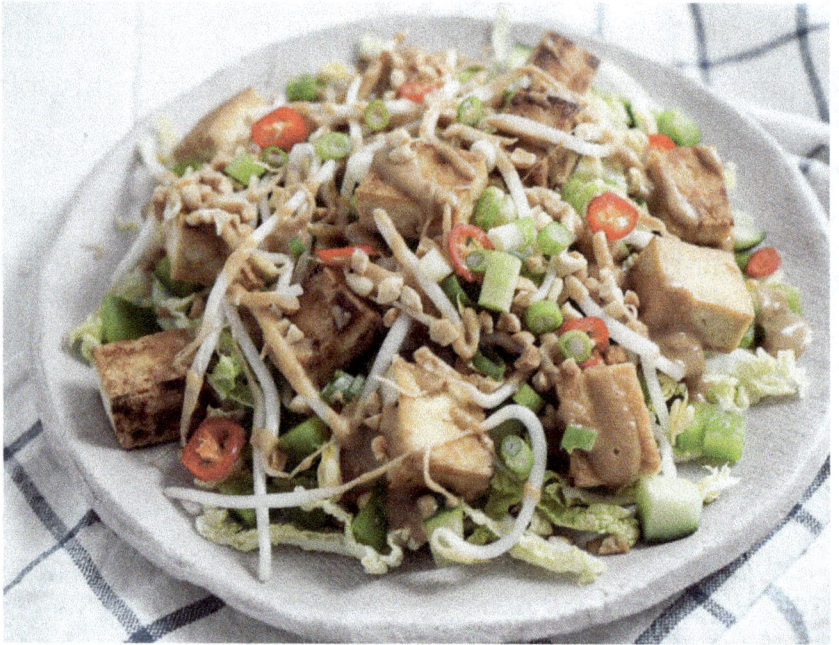

Kidney Beans, Quinoa, Vegetable and Salsa Bowl

Preparation time: 5 minutes Cooking time: 20 minutes Servings: 2

Ingredients:

For the Kidney Beans: 1 ½ cups cooked kidney beans 3/4 teaspoon salt 1 large tomato 3 cloves of garlic, peeled 1/2 teaspoon onion powder 1/2 inch piece of ginger 1/2 teaspoon paprika 1/2 teaspoon dried fenugreek leaves 1/3 teaspoon red chili powder 1/4 teaspoon turmeric 1 teaspoon coriander powder 1/2 teaspoon garam masala 1/2 teaspoon cumin powder 1 teaspoon lemon juice 1/2 cup water

For the Vegetables: Sliced roasted zucchini as needed Sliced roasted broccoli stems as needed Sliced radishes as needed Sliced lettuce as needed Mango salsa as needed

Directions:

Prepare the beans, and for this, place all the ingredients, except the first two ones, in a blender, pulse until smooth, then add this mixture into a saucepan and cook for 7 minutes over medium heat until thickened. Then stir in beans, season with salt, and cook for 12 minutes until beans are very tender. When done, place beans in a large bowl, top with vegetables and salsa, toss until mixed and serve

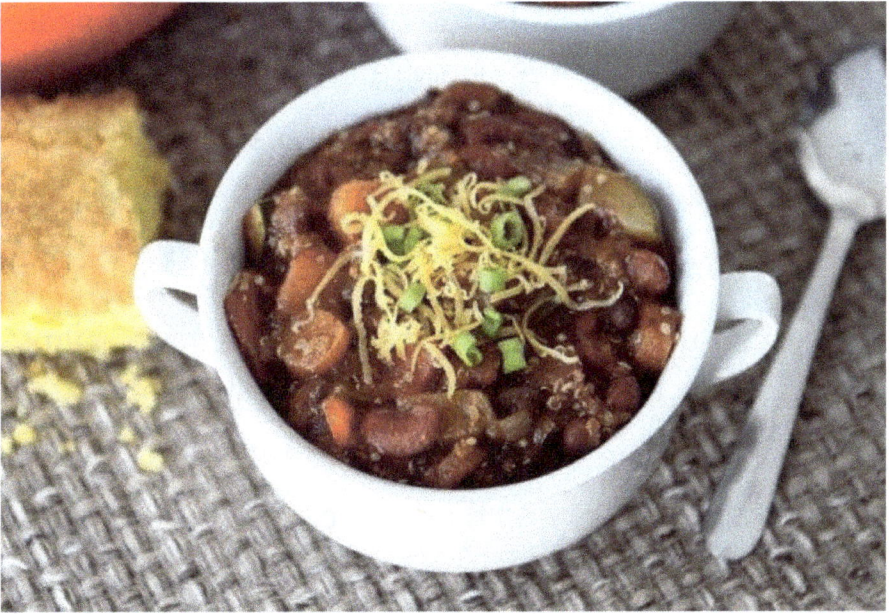

Rainbow Salad Bowl

Preparation time: 10 minutes Cooking time: 0 minute Servings: 4

Ingredients:

1 cup cooked quinoa 1 tablespoon hemp seeds 1 head of romaine lettuce, rib removed, leaves chopped 1/2 avocado, peeled, pitted, sliced ¼ of pickled red onion 1/2 cup diced cucumber ¼ cup pomegranate seeds ½ of lime, juiced 1/2 cup cilantro lime hummus

Directions:

Place all the ingredients except for lime juice, hummus, and hemp seeds in a bowl and toss until mixed. Place hummus in the middle, drizzle with lime juice, sprinkle with hemp seeds, and then serve.

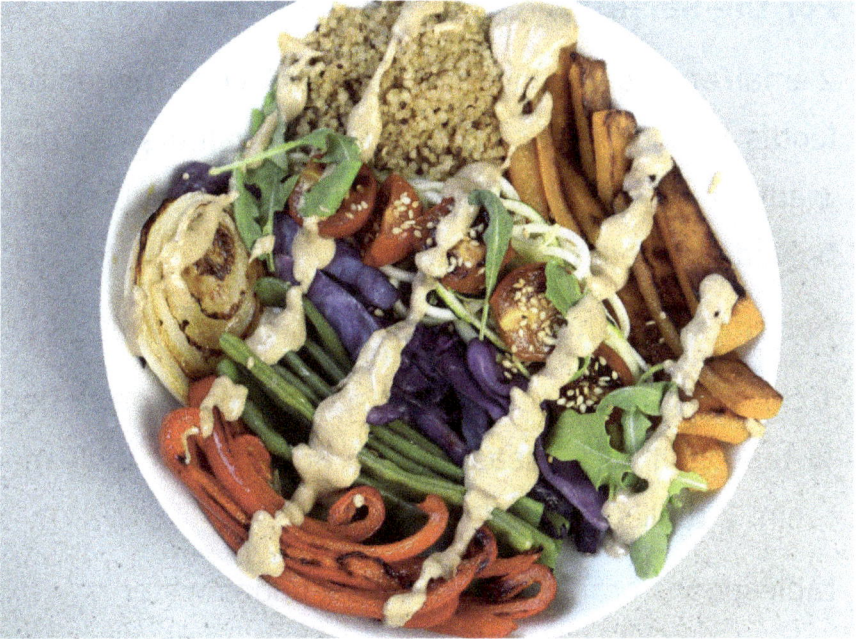

Lentil Salad With Spinach

Preparation time: 10 minutes Cooking time: 0 minute
Servings: 4

Ingredients:

For the Salad:

2 small apples, cut into small pieces 3 cups cooked brown lentils ½ cup fresh spinach 1/2 cup walnuts, chopped 1 medium avocado, pitted, cut into slices 1 pomegranate, halved, seeded, rinsed

For the dressing:

1 clove of garlic, peeled ¼ teaspoon ground black pepper ¼ teaspoon salt 2 teaspoons orange zest 3 tablespoons tahini 2 tablespoons olive oil 4

tablespoons orange juice 6 tablespoons water

Directions:

Prepare the dressing, and for this, place all of its ingredients in a food processor and pulse until smooth. Prepare the salad and for this, place all its ingredients in a bowl, toss until mixed, then drizzle with prepared dressing and stir until combined. Serve straight away.

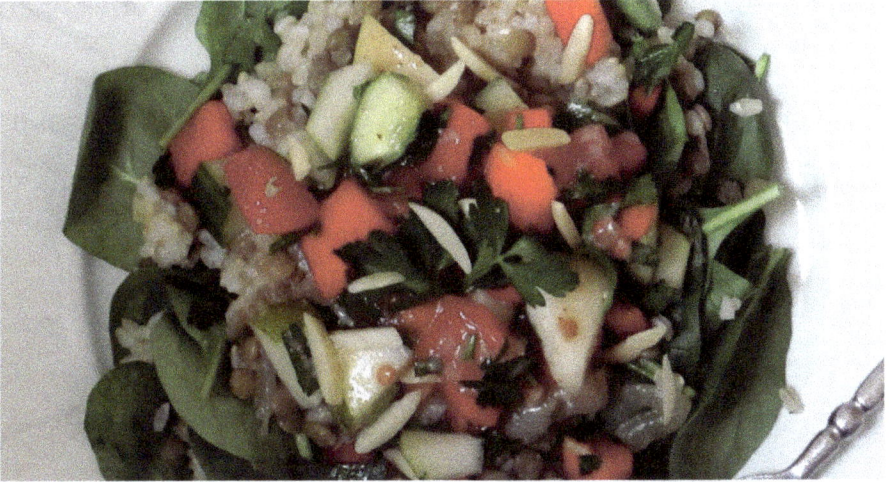

Grilled Corn Salad Bowl

Preparation time: 10 minutes Cooking time: 0 minute Servings: 4

Ingredients:

½ cup of beluga lentils, cooked 2 ears of fresh corn, grilled ½ cup pickled onions 1 medium avocado, peeled, sliced 1 green chili, chopped 2 cups arugula ¼ teaspoon ground black pepper 2/3 teaspoon salt 2 limes, juiced 4 tablespoons olive oil 10 basil leaves, chopped ¼ cup pine nuts, toasted

Directions: Place all the ingredients in the bowl, except for lime juice and oil, and stir until mixed. Drizzle with lime juice and oil, toss until mixed and serve.

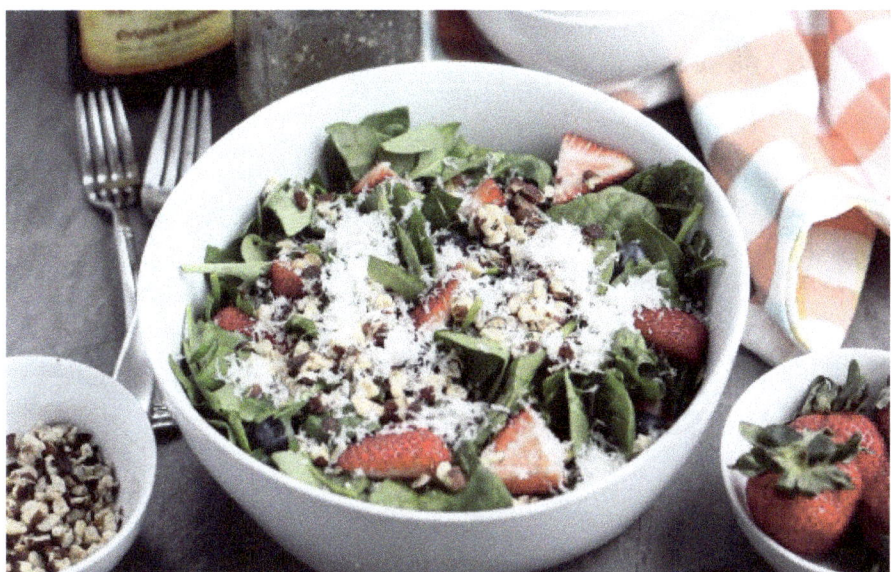

Roasted Butternut Squash Salad

Preparation time: 10 minutes Cooking time: 30 minutes

Servings: 4

Ingredients:

For the Dressing:

1/8 teaspoon salt

2 tablespoons lime juice

1 tablespoon olive oil

1 teaspoon sriracha

1/2 teaspoon honey

For the Salad:

4 cups arugula

1 pound butternut squash, peeled, cubed

1 1/2 teaspoons olive oil

3/4 cups cooked black beans

1/4 teaspoon ground black pepper

1/4 teaspoon salt

1/2 teaspoon ground cumin

1/4 cup pepitas, toasted

Directions:

Place squash cubes on a baking tray, drizzle with oil, season with salt, black pepper, and cumin, toss until coated and bakefor 30 minutes until roasted. Meanwhile, prepare the dressing and for this, place all of its ingredients in a bowl and whisk until smooth. When squash is done, let it cool for 10 minutes, then place it in a bowl along with remaining ingredients of the salad, drizzle with dressing and toss until mixed. Serve straight away.

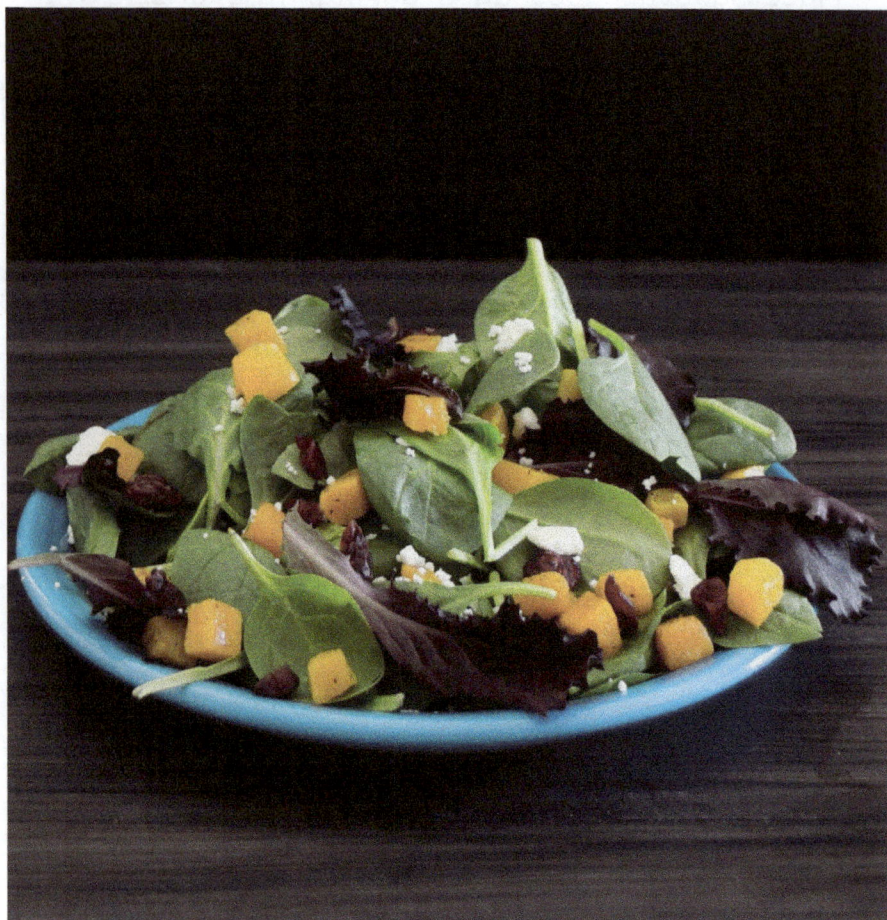

BBQ Chickpea Salad

Preparation time: 10 minutes Cooking time: 10 minutes Servings: 2

Ingredients:

2 cups cooked chickpeas 1 cup frozen corn kernel ¼ of medium red onion, sliced 1 cup cherry tomatoes, halved 6 cups chopped romaine lettuce 1 cup cucumber, sliced 6 Tablespoons Ranch Dressing 1/2 cup vegan BBQ sauce Lime wedges for garnish

Directions: Simmer chickpeas in the BBQ sauce for 10 minutes until chickpeas are glazed with it. Then divide remaining ingredients between two bowls, top with chickpeas, drizzle with dressing and serve with lime wedges.

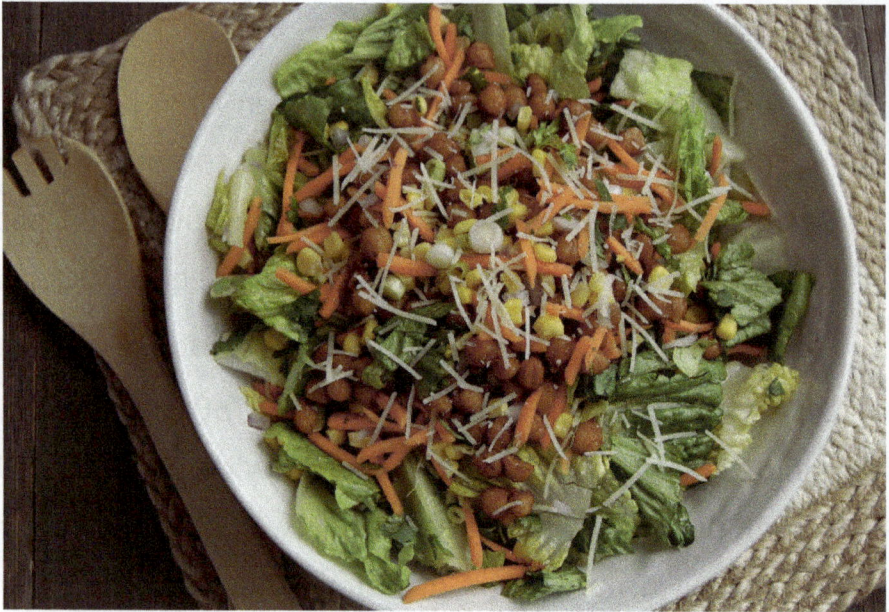

Butternut Squash Quinoa Salad

Preparation time: 10 minutes Cooking time: 25 minutes Servings: 4

Ingredients:

For the Salad: 1 cup quinoa, cooked 3 cups butternut squash, chopped 1/3 cup dried cranberries 1/3 cup chopped red onion 2/3 teaspoon salt 1/3 teaspoon ground black pepper 3 tablespoons toasted pumpkin seeds 1 tablespoon olive oil

For the Dressing: ½ teaspoon minced garlic 1/3 teaspoon salt 1/3 teaspoon ground black pepper 1 teaspoon honey 1/4 cup balsamic vinegar 1 teaspoon Dijon mustard 1/2 cup olive oil

Directions: Spread butternut squash on a baking sheet, drizzle with oil, season with black pepper and salt and bake for 25 minutes until roasted and tender. Meanwhile, prepare the dressing and for this, place all of its ingredients in a bowl and whisk until smooth. When done, let squash for 10 minutes, then place them in a bowl, add remaining ingredients for the salad in it, drizzle with dressing and toss until coated. Refrigerate the salad for a minimum of 2 hours and then serve.

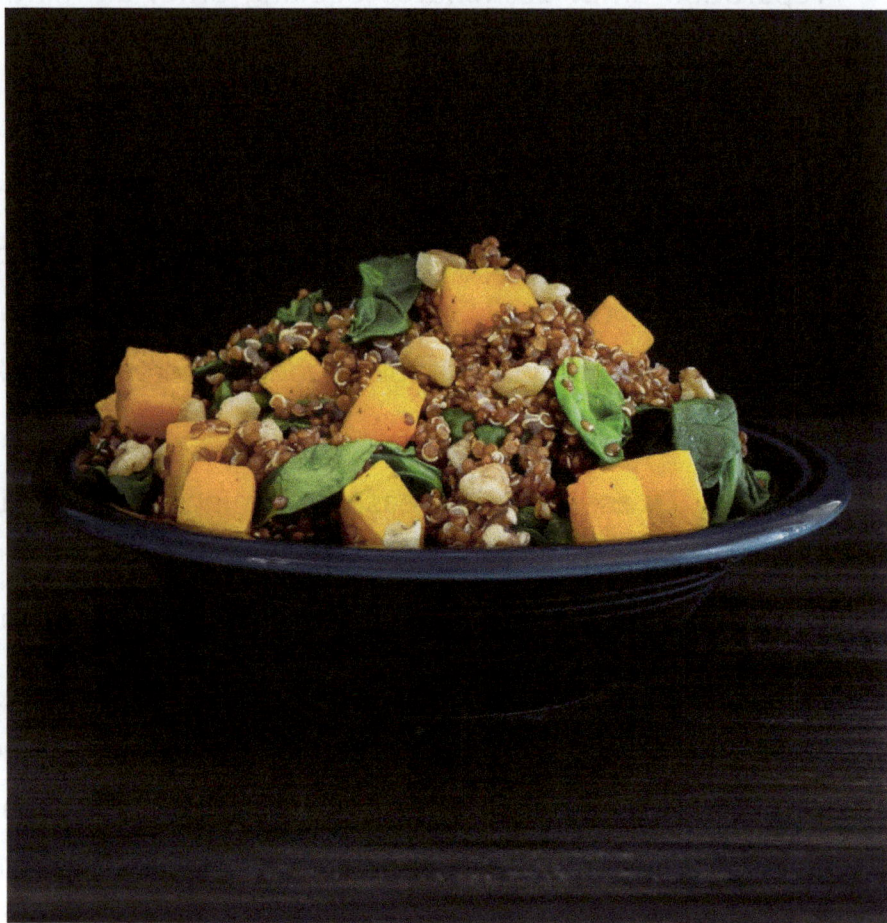

Cobb Salad

Preparation time: 10 minutes Cooking time: 0 minute Servings: 4

Ingredients:

For the Salad:

1/2 cup cooked red beans 1/2 cup cooked corn 1 medium head of romaine lettuce, shredded 1/2 cup chopped tempeh bacon 1/2 cup diced tomatoes 1/2 cup diced avocado 1/2 cup cashews, unsalted

For the Dressing:

1 teaspoon garlic powder 2 tablespoons lemon juice 3 tablespoons soy sauce 2 tablespoons cider vinegar 1/4 cup agave syrup 2 tablespoons Dijon mustard 1/4 cup olive oil 1/4 cup water

Directions:

Prepare the dressing, and for this, place all of its ingredients in a food processor and pulse until smooth. Place all the ingredients for the salad in a large dish, arrange each ingredients in a row, and then drizzle with prepared dressing. Serve straight away.

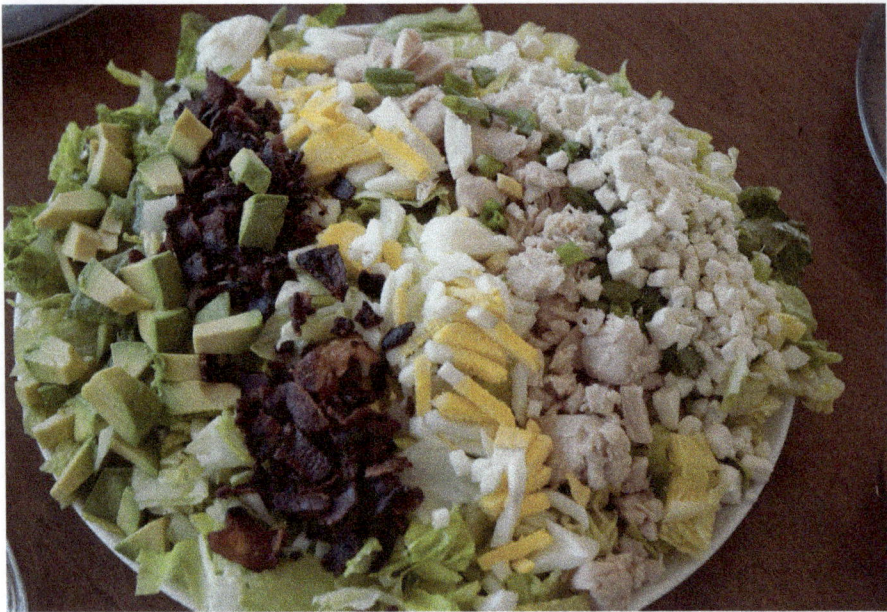

Vegan Caesar Salad

Preparation time: 10 minutes Cooking time: 30 minutes

Servings: 4

Ingredients:

½ cup chickpea croutons

10 ounces tofu, firmed, drain, dice

1 romaine lettuce, chopped

1 cup vegan Caesar dressing

¼ cup grated vegan Parmesan cheese

For the Dressing:

½ teaspoon garlic powder

½ teaspoon ground black pepper

½ teaspoon sweet paprika

½ teaspoon onion powder

½ teaspoon cumin

½ teaspoon dried thyme

3 tablespoons soy sauce

3 tablespoons water

Directions:

Place tofu pieces on a baking sheet lined with baking paper and then bake for 30 minutes at 390 degrees F until golden brown on all sides, turning halfway. Meanwhile, prepare the dressing and for this, place all of its ingredients in a bowl and whisk until smooth. When tofu has roasted, let it cool for 5 minutes, then add to the bowl along with remaining ingredients for the salad, drizzle with prepared dressing and toss until combined. Serve straight away.

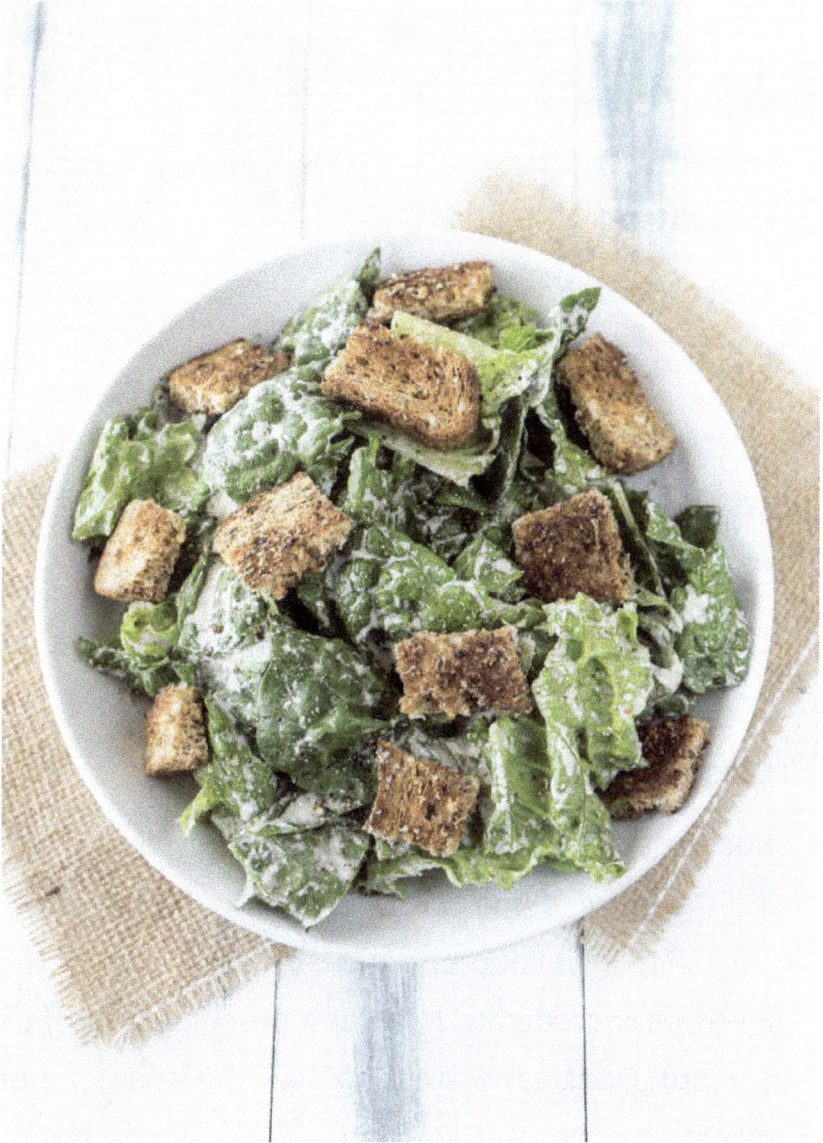

Vegan Chinese Salad

Preparation time: 10 minutes Cooking time: 0 minute Servings: 4

Ingredients:

For the Salad:

1 iceberg lettuce, chopped 1/4 cup soybean sprouts 2 carrots, peeled, julienned 1/4 cup agar, hydrated

For the Dressing:

1/4 teaspoon salt 1/4 cup coconut sugar 1 tablespoon olive oil 1/4 cup apple cider vinegar

Directions:

Soak agar in water until hydrated, then drain it and place it in a bowl along with remaining ingredients for the salad. Meanwhile, prepare the dressing and for this, place all of its ingredients in a food processor and pulse until smooth. Drizzle the dressing over the salad, stir until well mixed and then serve.

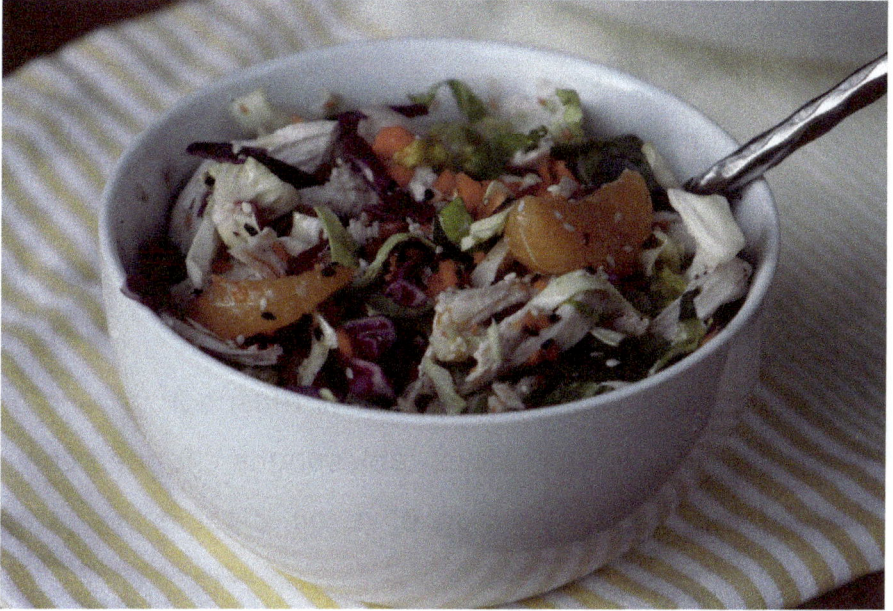

Heirloom Tomato Salad

Preparation time: 10 minutes Cooking time: 0 minute Servings: 6

Ingredients:

For the Salad:

1 pound heirloom tomatoes, cut into wedges ½ teaspoon salt ½ teaspoon ground black pepper ¼ cup basil leaves, for serving

For the Dressing:

2 cups grape tomatoes, halved ¼ teaspoon ground black pepper ½ teaspoon salt 2 tablespoons chopped chives 1 teaspoon honey 1/4 cup olive oil 2 tablespoons apple cider vinegar

Directions:

Prepare the dressing for this, whisk together honey, vinegar, oil, salt, and black pepper until combined, then add chives and tomatoes and toss until combined. Prepare the salad and for this, place tomatoes on a plate, season with salt and black pepper, drizzle with the dressing and top with basil. Serve straight away.

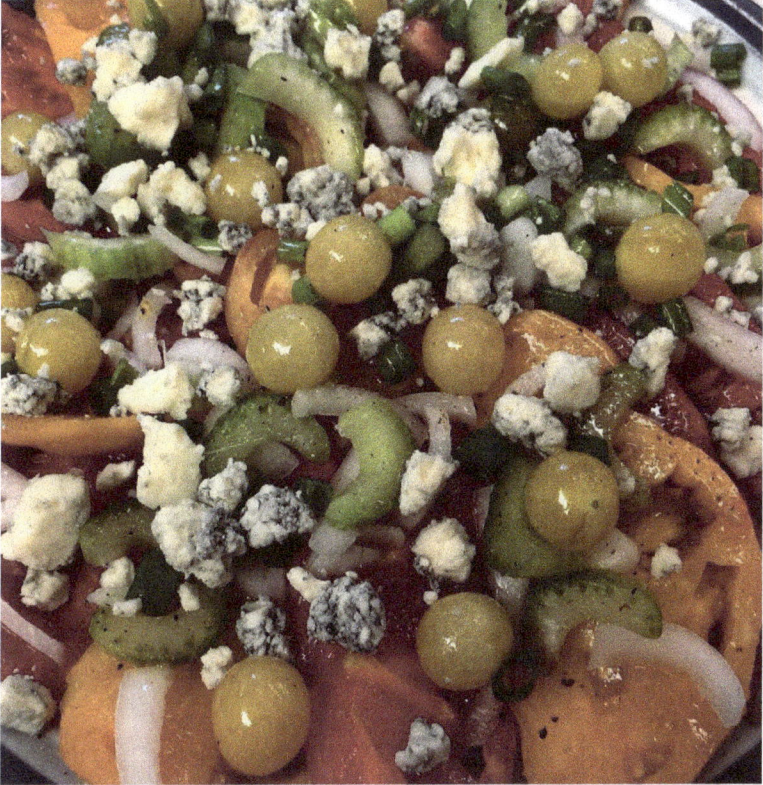

Zucchini Salad

Preparation time: 10 minutes Cooking time: 15 minutes
Servings: 4

Ingredients:

2 cups cubed zucchini 1 tablespoon chopped mint 1 small white onion, peeled, sliced ½ of a lemon, juiced 1 teaspoon minced garlic 2 tablespoons olive oil 1/8 teaspoon ground white pepper ¼ teaspoon salt 1/8 teaspoon ground turmeric 1/2 teaspoon ground cumin 7 saffron threads

Directions:

Take a skillet pan, place it over medium heat, add oil and when hot, add onion and garlic, and cook for 4 minutes until softened. Then add remaining ingredients, except for salt, black pepper, lime juice, and mint, stir until mixed and cook for 8 minutes until zucchini is tender-crisp. When done, let the salad cool for 10 minutes, then season with salt and black pepper, drizzle with lemon juice, sprinkle with mint and serve

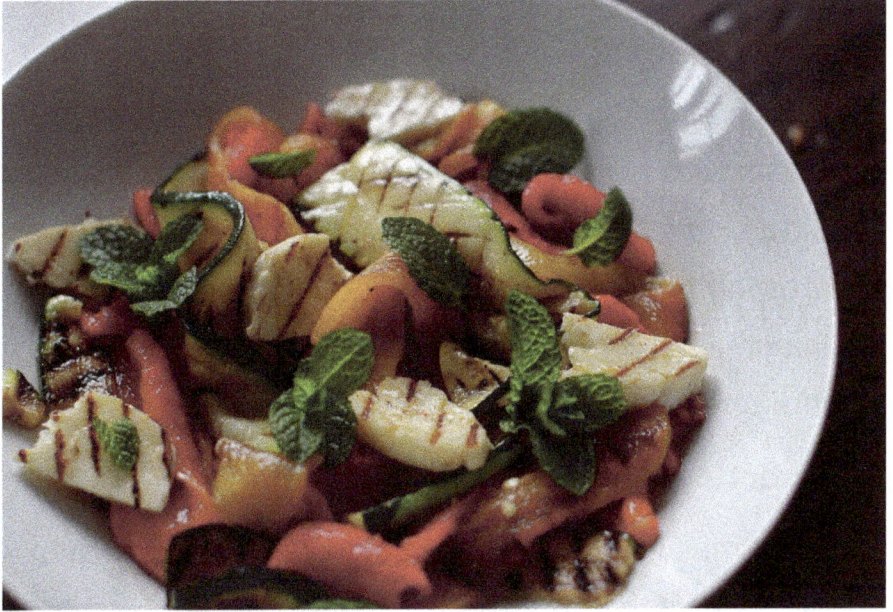

Beet, Mushroom and Avocado Salad

Preparation time: 15 minutes Cooking time: 20 minutes
Servings: 4

Ingredients:

8 ounces cooked beets, chopped 4 medium portobello mushroom caps 5 ounces baby kale 2 medium avocados, pitted, sliced 1 small shallot, peeled, chopped ¾ teaspoon salt ¼ teaspoon ground black pepper 1/4 cup lemon juice 3 tablespoons olive oil 2 sheets of matzo, cut into bite-size pieces

Directions:

Place mushroom caps on a baking sheet, spray them with oil, then season them with ½ teaspoon salt and bake for 20 minutes at 450 degrees F until tender. Place shallots in a small bowl, add black pepper and remaining salt, pour in oil and lemon juice and whisk until combined. Place kale and beets in a dish, drizzle with shallot mixture and toss until combined. When mushrooms have roasted, let them cool for 10 minutes, then slice them and to the kale mixture along with remaining ingredients. Toss until well combined and serve.

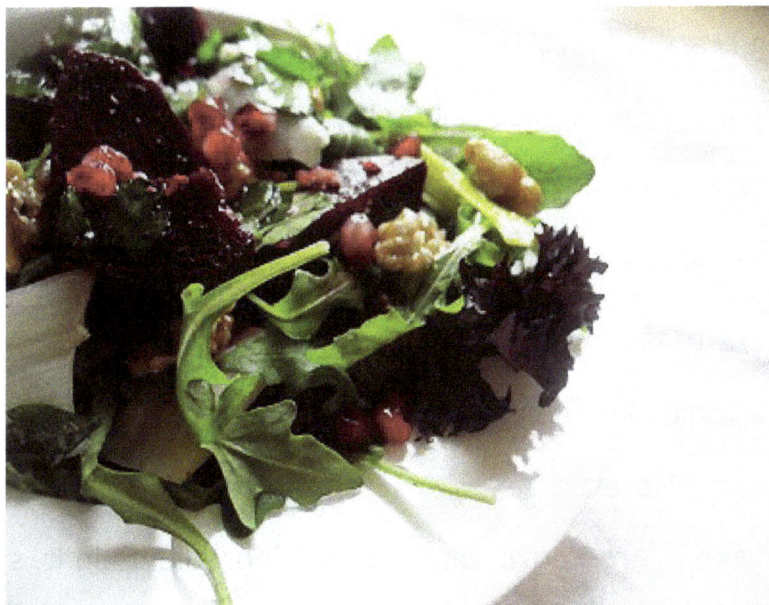

Tomato Basil Salad

Preparation time: 10 minutes Cooking time: 0 minute Servings: 4

Ingredients:

3 tablespoons chopped red onion

1 pound tomatoes, chopped

10 leaves of basil, cut into ribbons

1/4 teaspoon ground black pepper

1/2 teaspoon salt

2 tablespoons white balsamic vinegar

Directions:

Take a large bowl, place all the ingredients in it, stir until well combined, and then let it sit for 5 minutes. Refrigerate the salad for a minimum of 2 hours and then serve straight away.

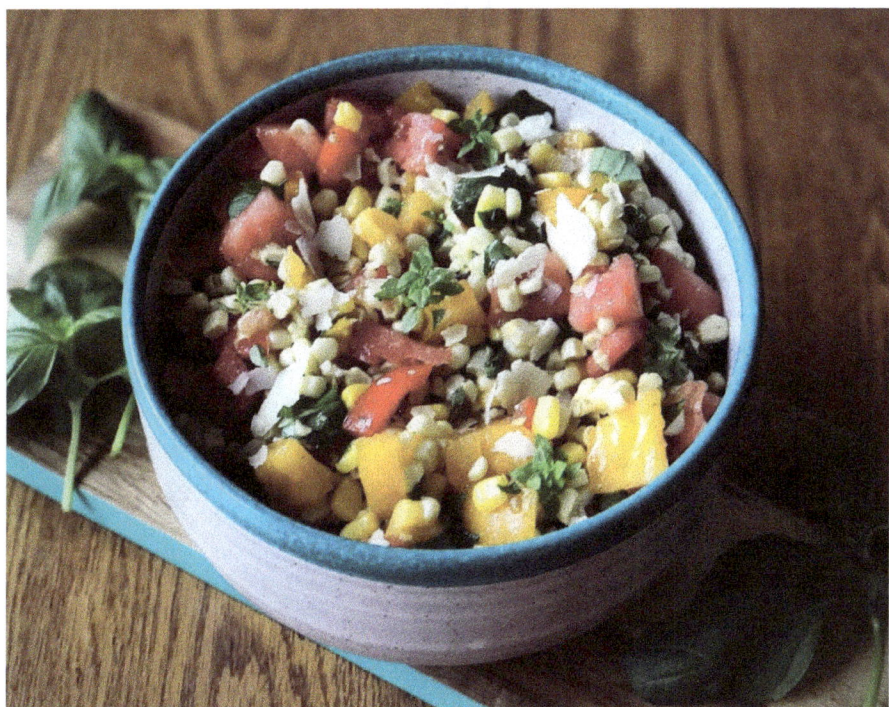

Sweet Potato and Cauliflower Salad

Preparation time: 10 minutes Cooking time: 30 minutes
Servings: 8

Ingredients:

For the Salad:

1 1/2 pound small sweet potatoes, peeled, cut into ½-inch wedges

2/3 cup pomegranate seeds

1 small head of cauliflower, cut into florets

8 cups mixed lettuces

1/2 teaspoon salt

1/4 teaspoon ground black pepper

3 tablespoons olive oil, divided

For the Dressing:

4 tablespoons olive oil, divided

1/2 teaspoon salt

1/4 teaspoon ground black pepper

3 tablespoons apple cider vinegar

Directions:

Take a baking sheet, place all the vegetables for the salad on it, drizzle with oil, season with salt and black pepper, toss until well coated, and then bake for 30 minutes at 425 degrees F until roasted. Meanwhile, prepare the dressing and for this, place all of its ingredients in a bowl and whisk until combined. When vegetables have roasted, let them cool for 10 minutes, then place them in a large bowl along with remaining ingredients for the salad, drizzle with the dressing and toss until coated. Serve straight away.

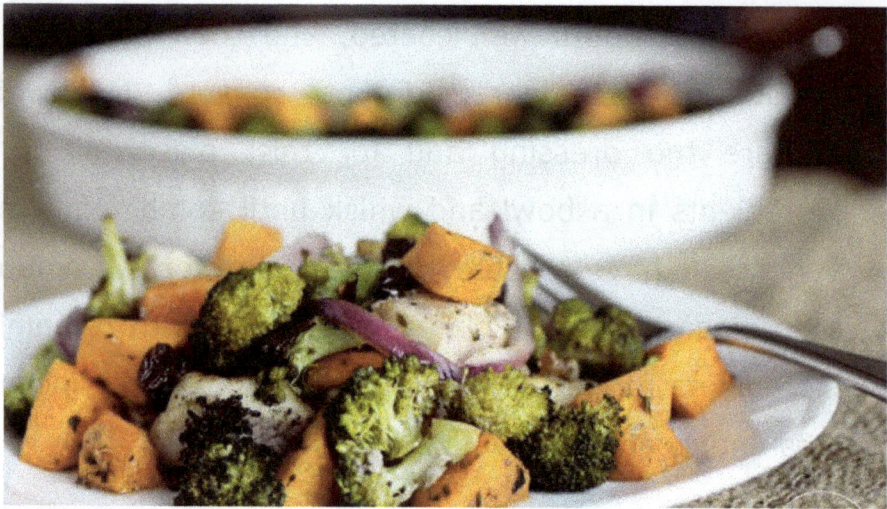

Fennel and Asparagus Salad

Preparation time: 10 minutes Cooking time: 8 minutes
Servings: 4

Ingredients:

For the Salad: 1 cup sliced asparagus, trimmed 1 large leek, white part sliced in circles only 1 medium avocado, pitted, sliced 2 cups thinly sliced fennel bulb, trimmed 3 tablespoons olive oil ¼ cup almonds, toasted

For the Dressing: 1 tablespoon thyme 2 tablespoons lemon juice ¾ teaspoon sea salt ½ teaspoon ground black pepper 1 teaspoon ground coriander 3 tablespoons olive oil

Directions:

Prepare the dressing and for this, place all of its ingredients in a bowl and whisk until combined. Sauté leeks in oil for 6 minutes or until it wilts and turns golden brown, then season with some salt and let it cool. Take a large bowl, place all the ingredients for the salad in it, except for almonds, drizzle with the salad dressing and toss until well coated. Top the salad with the almonds and then serve.

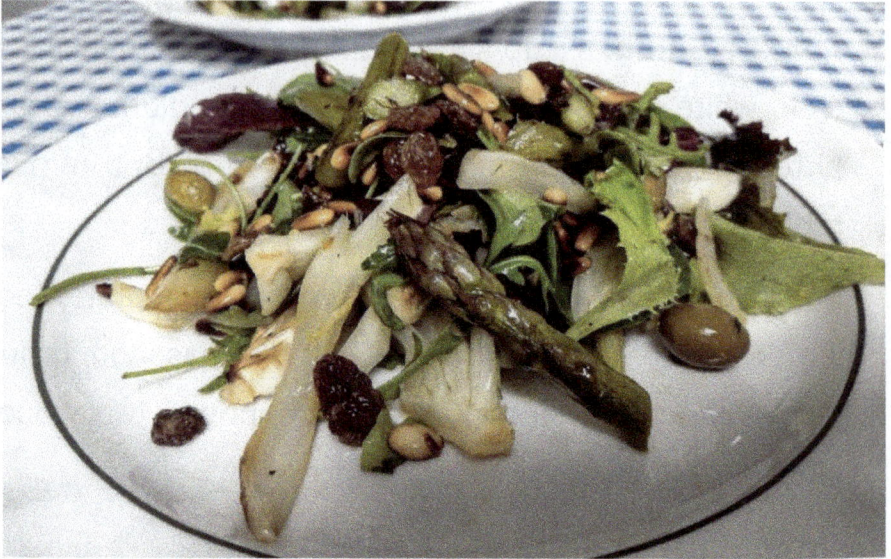

Thai Noodle Salad

Preparation time: 10 minutes Cooking time: 0 minute
Servings: 6

Ingredients:

For the Thai Peanut Sauce: 3 thin slices of ginger ½ teaspoon salt 3 tablespoon lime juice 1 clove of garlic, peeled 1 teaspoon cayenne pepper 2 tablespoons soy sauce ¼ cup peanut butter 3 tablespoons sesame oil ¼ cup of orange juice 3 tablespoons honey

For the Salad: 6 ounces brown rice noodles, cooked 4 cups mix of shredded cabbage, radish, and carrots 3 scallions, sliced 1 medium red bell pepper, peeled, sliced 1 tablespoon jalapeño, chopped ½ bunch of cilantro, chopped ½ cup roasted peanuts, crushed

Directions:

Prepare the sauce, and for this, place all of its ingredients in a blender and pulse until smooth. Take a large bowl, place all the ingredients for the salad in it, except for almonds, top with prepared sauce and toss until well coated. Top the salad with almonds and then serve straight away.

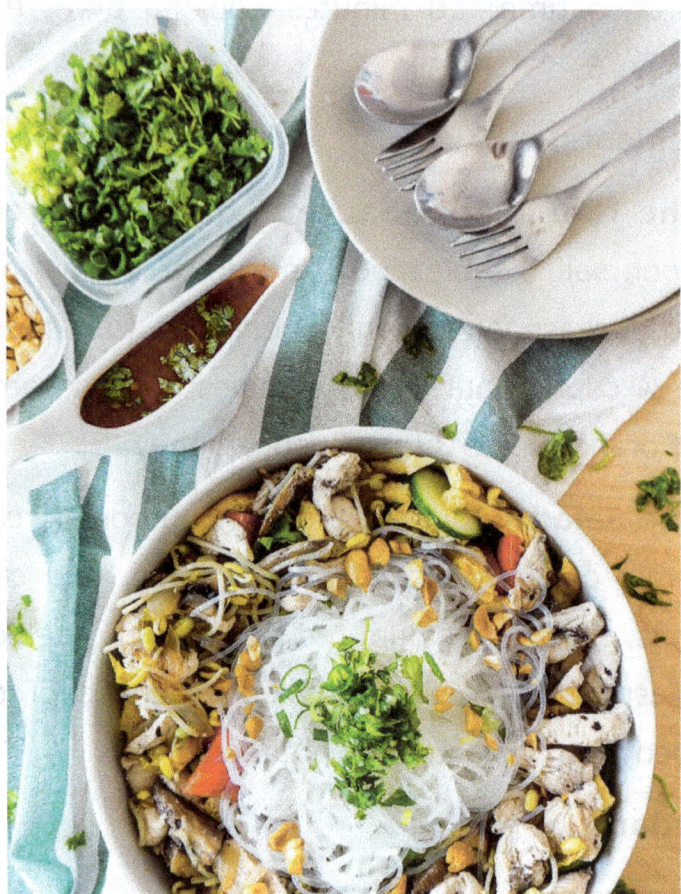

Cherry Tomato and Tofu Salad

Preparation time: 10 minutes Cooking time: 0 minute Servings: 2

Ingredients:

For the Salad: 2 slices of tofu 1 cup cherry tomatoes, halved 1 teaspoon sesame seeds

For the Dressing: 2 teaspoons soy sauce ¼ teaspoon ground black pepper ¼ teaspoon of sea salt 1 teaspoon sherry vinegar 1 teaspoon toasted sesame oil 2 tablespoons olive oil

Directions: Prepare the dressing and for this, place all of its ingredients in a small bowl and whisk until smooth. Place cherry tomatoes in a bowl, drizzle with dressing, toss until well coated and sprinkle with sesame seeds. Prepare the salad and for this, place tofu slices on a plate, top with tomato mixture and serve straight away.

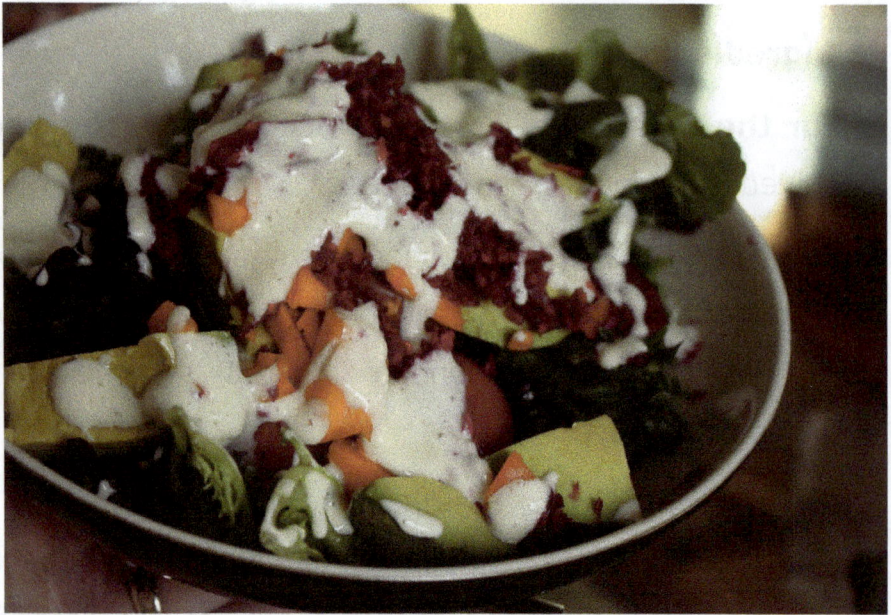

Cabbage and Mango Slaw

Preparation time: 20 minutes Cooking time: 0 minute Servings: 4

Ingredients:

1 jalapeno, chopped

3 cups shredded cabbage

¼ cup sliced red onion

1 large mango, destoned, cubed

½ cup chopped cilantro

½ teaspoon salt

1 orange, juiced, zested

2 teaspoons olive oil

1 lime, juiced, zested

Directions: Take a large bowl, place all the ingredients in it, and toss until well coated. Let the salad refrigerate for 15 minutes and then serve.

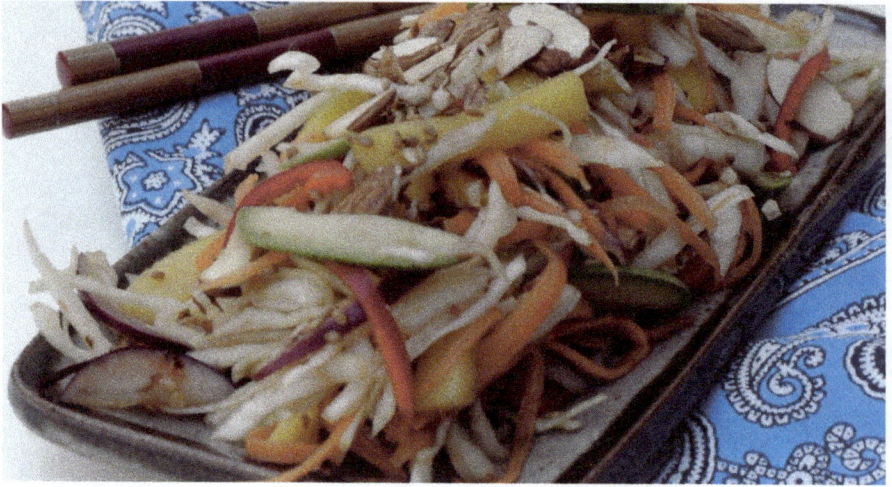

www.ingramcontent.com/pod-product-compliance
Lightning Source LLC
Chambersburg PA
CBHW050754030426
42336CB00012B/1813